GET HEALTHY
AND
LOSE WEIGHT

HOW TO FORM THE HABITS FOR

HEALTHY EATING AND A HEALTHY LIFESTYLE

By Ron & Julie Meiss

GET HEALTHY AND LOSE WEIGHT

Title: Get Healthy And Lose Weight
Subtitle: How to Form the Habits for Healthy Eating and a Healthy Lifestyle
Authors: Ron & Julie Meiss

Description: 15 years of independent research by the authors has clarified the critical habits of eating and drinking that most often leads to a condition of optimal health. This is not just another diet plan. This guidebook has been written in a manner that introduces the 10 habits of healthy eating in a style that facilitates daily learning by the reader. The healthy eating principles produce the ability to lose weight and a continuing healthy lifestyle.

Keywords: How Get Healthy, Lose Weight, Healthy Lifestyle, Eating Habits, Weight Loss, Diet Plan

Published by: The Center for Nutritional Science
Publishing website: www.gethealthyandloseweight.com

Cover design: Rick Hubbard Consulting – www.riverjumping.com

Cover art description: The design of the cover art is based upon the 2011 graphic from the USDA which depicts the current description of the food guide pyramid. The edition is titled MyPlate.

ISBN-13:ISBN-13: 978-1466374515

ISBN-10: 1466374519

DEDICATION

This book is dedicated to the memory of Ann Marie.

She lived this way for 91 years.

DISCLAIMER

The authors and publisher specifically disclaim all responsibility for any liability, loss, or risk, personal or otherwise, which is incurred as a consequence, directly or indirectly, of the use and application of any of the contents of this publication. This publication contains the opinions and ideas of its authors and editors. It is intended to provide helpful and informative material on the subjects addressed in the publication. It is sold with the understanding that the authors and publisher are not engaged in rendering medical, health, or any kind of personal professional services in this plan. The reader should consult his or her medical, health, or other competent professional before adopting any of the suggestions in this plan or drawing inferences from it.

FOREWORD

It all began in the Summer of 1994. One of our team members (Ron) was introduced to a California company that had just published a weight loss program. The exciting part was that it worked for all of us and the enthusiasm that we felt caused some of us to really become interested in this idea of **healthy weight** and created the desire to learn why some people were successful and others struggled. This momentum led to the official creation two years later of what is now our Center For Nutritional Science team.

Our research and publishing was in full swing by September of 1996 and we haven't looked back since. We've kept up on all of the latest medications and all of the many types of "nutra-ceuticals" that have been introduced in the marketplace. We've worked with more than 20 different companies, always searching for the very best answers for people who needed to release those unwanted pounds and inches.

This book is the result of those many efforts over the past 15 years. **We've learned a lot and have had to unlearn even more.** Our experience is that there is so much confusion surrounding this topic, we've had to keep our minds open and be willing to realize that much of what we believed was really just a bunch of myths and lies that had been accepted, often for the wrong reasons. We have been left with ten simple truths that we now share with you as The 10 Habits. Please know two things as you begin:

1. The Premise: You will soon become aware that we truly believe in the premise that it is far more effective to strive to get healthy first and then to lose weight. We have helped thousands of people lose weight. Frankly, it's not that difficult when you understand these principles. The challenge is to maintain a healthy weight. The good news is that there is a credible answer to that issue as well. We believe if St. Francis of Assisi was with us today, he would say: "Seek first to get healthy, then to lose weight."

2. The Essentials: Air, water, food, movement, and rejuvenation. We do not claim that we discovered the five essentials. After all, they are eternal components. We are excited that we have been able to combine all five in this collection of habits and offer you a total program of optimal health. Air is the most abundant and must be constantly replenished. Water makes up roughly two-thirds of the body and is also refreshed on a regular basis. Much of this learning is focused on food, the macro-nutrients and the micro-nutrients that make up the third of the essentials. Movement, often referred to as exercise is the fourth and rejuvenation is the fifth. Learned as a total package, these essentials are the foundation of what we refer to as Maximum Health. We are excited that you have chosen to seek the answers.

The Team at the Center for Nutritional Science

THE 10 HABITS TO
GET HEALTHY AND LOSE WEIGHT

HABIT 1: FOCUS ON YOUR WHY

HABIT 2: HYDRATE PROPERLY

HABIT 3: BREATHE EFFECTIVELY

HABIT 4: PLAN TO SUCCEED

HABIT 5: NOURISH WITH REAL FOOD

HABIT 6: MOVE TO ACTIVATE YOUR METABOLISM

HABIT 7: REFRESH TO STRENGTHEN YOUR COMMITMENT

HABIT 8: FUEL WITH PROTEIN FOR STRENGTH

HABIT 9: FUEL WITH CARBOHYDRATES FOR ENERGY

HABIT 10: FUEL WITH LIPIDS FOR NORMAL BODY FUNCTIONS

Ron & Julie Meiss

TABLE OF CONTENTS

Ron & Julie Meiss

PARTNER

As you begin to learn and implement the ideas in this guidebook you will experience several different lessons for each of the 10 Habits to Health. This is the first step you will take as you learn some new ideas and behaviors that will improve your health and make it possible for you to lose those unwanted pounds. Here's the best part: **you don't have to do it alone!**

We have worked with thousands of people over the past 15 years and have found that it works so much better when you learn this system with another person who will help "keep it moving and on target". Here's how it works…

1. Visit our website at www.gethealthyandloseweight.com

2. Select the header that is marked *Contact Us*

3. Enter the word **Partner** in the subject box

4. Please enter a message telling us when you first started the program and a little bit about your reason WHY. We'll provide the guidelines that we suggest you follow to select a helpful partner

5. We will also send you a copy of our informative guidebook titled, *Becoming a Healthy Weight Partner*

6. We promise you that it is that simple. We will do whatever it takes to help to help you succeed. That means that your Partner information is offered to you free of any charge or obligation

7. Please contact us at any time using the above directions

WELCOME

We welcome you on the journey to learn the habits that will lead to a healthy lifestyle and will assist you as you reach and maintain your lifetime healthy weight. Let's take a few minutes to focus on a clear picture of your reason for this decision. We have worked with thousands of people over the past 15 years and each has started with a definite purpose. We'll begin by developing a clear picture of your reason why.

This guidebook is the result of those many years of study, research, and much trial and error, as the founders of the Center for Nutritional Science have sought to better understand the issues of health and weight. We have spent time with more than 4000 people who were dealing with a variety of health issues. We have completed studies with 22 different product companies and nine very creative fitness companies.

This healthy eating plan has been created as a result of asking questions about some important health issues:

- What does it mean to be healthy?

- Are most people generally healthy?

- How much control do we have over our health?

- Can I count on new drugs and medications to help improve my health?

- Will the health care system be able to meet future needs?

- What is the overall quality of health care in our country?

- What impact do healthy habits have on my need for other healthcare services?

- Am I healthy? Is my family healthy?

- What improvements can I make in taking care of myself?

- How important is it for me to develop healthy habits?

These are questions each one of us needs to learn to answer for ourselves. We want to help you find the best possible answers. We start with this premise: **given your genetic coding at birth – your health is largely a result of your daily habits and choices.**

Og Mandino, the most widely-read self help author of all time and a very dear friend of ours always said, "Choice! The key is choice. You have options. You need not spend your life wallowing in failure, ignorance, grief, poverty, shame and self-pity. There is a better way to live." Unfortunately, many do not find it. We won't spend a lot of time on all of the details. We're all bombarded with the news reports of the issues of heart disease, diabetes, and other factors known as the Metabolic Syndrome. One of the biggest factors that emerges during the battle to stay free of these problems is maintaining a healthy weight.

Reputable studies suggest that more than 80% of the people who experience some success in their weight loss efforts, re-gain the lost pounds and inches over the next 3-5 years, usually adding at least an additional 4-5%. An acquaintance who weighed 217 pounds, dieted down to 189, and now about 6 years later weighs 228. If the goal is only to lose weight, it'll be back with a vengeance. Our objective is to get healthy and then learn habits that will lead to fat loss.

Why? Of the thousands of people that we've worked with during the past 15 years, most of them found us as they searched for answers related to their problems with body weight and excess fat. The most powerful thing we learned from them is that in order to achieve any amount of success on this journey, we must keep a constant focus on our "Why."

Spend some time now to consider your "Why." Get that awareness firmly planted in your thought process. We'll complete a worksheet in just a moment and then begin each week for the first four weeks with an exercise devoted to re-visiting that focus.

I (Julie) am a small person. I have had some health challenges in my life, but weight has not been an issue - until my early 50's. I experienced the normal changes that a woman expects at that point in her life, and I became increasingly aware of the added fat (nearly 20 extra pounds) accumulating around my midsection and my hips. At a Christmas dinner in 2009, I voiced my frustration to Ron (my future husband) who proceeded to ask me if it was strong enough to be my "Why." I agreed that it was, focused carefully on the eating plan in this book, and "released" the extra pounds before Easter. No crazy diet, no mad exercising, no goofy stimulants or extra supplements … just a daily discipline to the healthy eating plan. I have easily maintained that comfortable 107-109 pounds since.

Discipline creates freedom. We have learned some powerful principles during our years of working with clients who wanted to achieve a healthy weight. The most powerful is that Discipline creates freedom. How can *discipline* create freedom? It seems paradoxical but let's consider it.

One of the steps that we encourage before beginning the turnaround is that you listen to our audio recording titled "the Myths, Lies, and Hidden Traps that make us fat". It's available to you at www.gethealthyandloseweight.com. One of the hidden traps is described as **lack of proper hydration.** A challenge for many people who are trying to learn this eating plan is to learn a way to hydrate properly each day. This is only one discipline. Those who achieve the best results, learn several disciplines along the way, and then benefit from the **freedom** from worry over whether they've had enough to drink each day.

Here's how the hydration discipline works: You will learn quickly that it is important to begin your morning with a glass of room temperature water within the first hour of waking. The discipline required is to form the habit of drawing the glass of water each evening before retiring, and leaving it in a place where you will definitely see it the next morning. Rather than worry about remembering to have your water in the morning, put it in your daily plan to prepare the beverage the evening before.

A similar principle applies to eating every 3 hours and remembering to have two snacks on hand for each day. Those are examples of the habits or disciplines that will be developed in the coming weeks.

Let's face it.....the food and beverage companies and even the weight-loss industry do not have anything to gain by helping us succeed. The growers and the manufacturers of the food products make more profits when we continue to overeat and drink sweetened drinks and then, literally, get addicted to this unhealthy way of eating. This may sound harsh, but get serious ... your success is up to you and it will be based on your ability to learn what is in this guidebook and then apply it on a daily basis.

On the following pages are some **worksheets** to help you analyze where you are now. **The** *What is Your Why ?* **worksheet** helps you identify what can motivate you to develop the needed disciplines. The Healthy Lifestyle Worksheet helps you identify the areas where you need to develop the disciplines that bring the improvement you desire. When you have completed these two worksheets you should know the "Why" and the "What." The rest of the book will help you with "How" and "When." This will include a Detailed Daily Plan and a day-by-day guide to help you get healthy and lose weight.

WHERE'S THE EATING PLAN?

You may be asking, "Where's the eating plan?" You will soon realize that there is no rigid list. You see, changing habits takes time. You do it one step **at** a time, one day at a time. Our purpose is to help you establish sustainable habits so that the changes feel natural. We're not talking about quick weight loss as much as we are about a healthy, sustainable weight. While there is no master list, there is a **Sample Eating Plan** in just a few pages.

For the most part the plan for successful change is delivered one day at a time. You will learn how this works in Week 1 – Day 1. There will be guidelines each day to help you focus and commit. To encourage you to be accountable and keep going, there is a journal for each day as you begin to learn the habits. We'll talk more about the journal on the first day of the program.

It's a change of lifestyle so you're healthier. It's not a crash-diet like others you've tried before. To get started, fill out the following worksheets and then start on Week 1 – Day 1.

LET'S GET STARTED ON THE JOURNEY TO BETTER HEALTH!

WHAT IS YOUR WHY WORKSHEET

Through the years people have shared with us the reasons why they want to make a change. We have identified the top ten reasons they give. Read and consider each reason; then select the top two or three that apply to you. Perhaps you have a different reason; include it on lines 11 or 12.

CHECK THE REASONS THAT APPLY TO YOU.

1._____ I am becoming concerned about my health.

2._____ I really don't like the way I look.

3._____ I would like to lose about _____ pounds.

4._____ My favorite clothes don't fit well any longer.

5._____ My doctor has advised me to _____.

6._____ I just want to feel better.

7._____ I am always tired; I have so little energy.

8._____ I want to do this for_____ i.e. spouse, children, etc.

9._____ I want to look good for an important upcoming event .

10._____ I want to improve the quality of my life.

11._____ _____. (Other)

12._____ _____. (Other)

Describe how you will look and feel when you accomplish your goal.

Ron & Julie Meiss

HEALTHY LIFESTYLE WORKSHEET

Rate each of the following statements using a 0-5 score shown below. At the end of each section add the total for that section and record it.

| Most Days: 5 | Many Days: 4 | Some Days: 3 | Very Seldom: 2 | Never: 0 |

BREATHE

_____ I am able to avoid being around cigarette smoke

_____ I take time throughout the day to breathe deeply

_____ I relax and lower my stress with rhythmic breathing

_____ I can avoid smog or polluted air

_____ I have healthy lungpower

Total Score for breathing: _____

HYDRATE

_____ I drink several glasses of pure water daily

_____ I avoid beverages while I'm eating

_____ I drink only small amounts of sweetened beverages

_____ I limit my caffeine intake

_____ I get liquid from eating fresh fruits and vegetables

Total Score for hydration: _____

NOURISH

_____ I get plenty of protein throughout the day

_____ I make it a point to eat smaller amounts, more often

_____ I enjoy a healthy breakfast each morning

_____ I avoid processed and packaged foods

_____ I eat slowly and chew my food thoroughly

Total Score for eating: _____

MOVE

_____ I take time throughout the day to stretch

_____ I get up and move around, periodically

_____ I get some exercise

_____ I enjoy a favorite sport or activity

_____ I am about as active as I can be

Total Score for movement: _____

REFRESH

_____ I wake rested and ready for the day

_____ I get enough sleep

_____ I am able to manage my level of stress

_____ I have plenty of energy

_____ I sleep on a good, comfortable bed

Total Score for rejuvenation: _____

WHAT DOES THE SCORE MEAN?

21-25: Keep it up ... look for small signs of progress

16-20: At least one statement needs improvement

11-15: Average ... but who wants to be average

0-10: Clearly room for improvement

SAMPLE HEALTHY LIFESTYLE PLAN

6:30 to 7 AM: Wake up and enjoy some water

Before you put any coffee, tea, or food of any type into your body, it's best to first *break your fast* with a glass of room temperature water. When you sleep, your body isn't just fasting from food but from water too.

7 AM: Short walk

This is an ideal fat-burning energizer. Aim for a light boost of cardio soon after you wake up and before you eat, such as a walk with the dog. Try running The idea is to fit in some easy activity and then eat within an hour of waking.

7:30 AM: Breakfast

We are going to learn a lot about this most important meal of the day. We will focus on enjoying a blended breakfast: one that contains protein and fiber.

Here's the key: Whatever you do, don't just sip coffee all morning and wait to eat until lunch. You'll be so hungry, you won't make healthy choices.

9 AM to 11 AM: Morning beverage

We're going to learn that we do well with about five servings of beverage a day, and it's better to sip a little all day long instead of chugging a giant glass when you suddenly feel parched. It's all about keeping the body properly hydrated throughout the day.

10 to 10:30 AM: Stretch and snack

If your work keeps you, desk-bound, it is important to get up every hour or so and move around. Eat every 3 hours to keep energy up and avoid mealtime binges. Try an apple with a string cheese or a handful of nuts.

12:30 PM: Water and some light activity

Finish your morning glass, refill it, and drink some more good clear water. Then get up and stretch at your desk. It jump starts your digestive system.

1 to 1:30 PM: Mid-day meal

This is a great time for a blended meal and/or a serving from one of the three "S" options. Enjoy Soup, Salad, or a healthy Sandwich.

2 PM: Beverage and a walk

Doing this now will help you make a sensible choice when those afternoon cravings strike. Get outside if you can, especially if you didn't go out for lunch .The fresh air and sunshine will boost your spirits and stop you from overeating because of a bad mood.

3:30 to 4 PM: Afternoon snack

Almost everyone needs to snack sometime between lunch and dinner. Try a 6-ounce yogurt (the natural milk sugars help with sweet cravings) and a handful of high-fiber cereal. Or, have a small banana with a tablespoon of peanut or almond butter.

Bonus Tip: Let your appetite be your guide. If you had a big lunch, you may only need a small nibble. If you plan to hit the gym after work, you may want to eat more or save some of your snack until an hour or so before your workout.

6 to 7 PM: Walk or work out

If you didn't walk in the morning, now is a good time for some exercise. When you're home waiting before dinner is often when the munchies happen. Keep moving with some type of pre-dinner activity.

7:30 PM: Dinner

Start this meal off with soup to help you slow down, and to get your digestive juices flowing. Studies show that people who do this, end up eating less overall. Have a cup of a low-fat broth-based kind like minestrone, miso, or gazpacho.

For the main meal select a 3-4 ounce serving of your favorite protein (Salmon, chicken, or lean meat, for instance), a colorful salad and some lightly-steamed vegetables.

10:30 to 11 PM: Time for bed

Aim for 7 to 8 hours of sleep a night; less than that, and you up your risk for a host of health problems, including weight gain, diabetes, high blood pressure, and more.

You'll be less likely to feel overly tired, frazzled, and you'll be less likely to overeat the next day. Give yourself plenty of time to wind down with a calming routine, such as a bath, shower, or reading in bed.

PART I

WEEK 1 - WEEK 4

THE FIRST 7 HABITS

HABIT 1: FOCUS ON YOUR WHY

HABIT 2: HYDRATE PROPERLY

HABIT 3: BREATHE EFFECTIVELY

HABIT 4: PLAN TO SUCCEED

HABIT 5: NOURISH WITH REAL FOOD

HABIT 6: MOVE TO ACTIVATE YOUR METABOLISM

HABIT 7: REFRESH TO STRENGTHEN YOUR COMMITMENT

Ron & Julie Meiss

Week 1 – Day 1

"I am committed to developing a plan for health eating."

HABIT 1: FOCUS ON YOUR WHY

We have an incredible opportunity here. We are committed to working together to help you take what has become a complex and confusing activity that you do several times each day, and turn it into something that makes sense and is "good for you". We are talking about healthy eating (and drinking) so that you can learn to attain and maintain a healthy weight and so you can have plenty of energy to accomplish everything you choose to do as a part of your active life.

By focusing on learning and practicing these daily habits, you will discover that this does not have to be such a confusing issue and that you can feel better each day and avoid much (maybe all) of the sickness that seems to "go around".

Just like everything in life, this will work for you if you focus and "take it one day at a time." Even though there are eight weeks of training in this guidebook, we ask you to put today's date on the journal page and to simply take one step at a time. Let's face it…you're busy, you don't really want to have to think about this "stuff", and your eating habits have been developed over many years.

We'll get to the point of healthy eating and drinking if we simply follow each step for a day, and then continue to implement that step and improve each day. By the time we put all of these steps and habits together, it will all make sense and you will find that you actually enjoy your new lifestyle.

Read and think about focusing on the benefits of eating well. Then concentrate on the commitment statement that is actually the very first line of every lesson, write it down where you will see it throughout the day, and say it several times. You will probably have it memorized by the end of the day. Practice the simple activities and you are on your way to a "lifetime of healthy eating". You may or may not add years to your life, but you will certainly add "life" to your years.

ABOUT THE JOURNAL PAGES

Make the choice to journal your experience today and along the way. It will help you focus; focus and you'll learn and develop healthy habits.

Start by taking some time to think about some of the reasons why you would like to learn healthy eating. Be real clear about the benefits for following through with this decision. Continually focus on your reasons why. You are tapping into your greatest power … the power to choose.

◆———————————————————◆

GET HEALTHY JOURNAL

Date:

"I am committed to developing a plan for health eating."

HABIT 1: FOCUS ON YOUR WHY.

One thing I really want to learn is:

One thing I think I do well is:

One thing I want to focus on changing is:

ADMIT YOUR DESIRE TO CHANGE … CHOOSE TO FOCUS

WEEK 1 – DAY 2

"I begin each day with a glass of clean water
and stay hydrated all day."

HABIT 2: HYDRATE PROPERLY

Whenever we look at any type of plan to improve our health, drinking plenty of healthy beverages is one of the first requirements. You've probably asked "Is it really that necessary?" The short answer is: Absolutely!

In terms of sheer volume, water is the second most abundant element that the body requires for nutrition. Air – oxygen – is the first. You probably remember learning in school that the human body is anywhere from 55% to as much as 78% water, depending on body size. That means that roughly two thirds of your body weight consists of water; which makes it the single largest component.

Our objective here is to take a look at the facts, and quickly translate the facts into practical steps we can learn, understand, and apply. You lose roughly 50% of your body weight in ounces of liquid each day or more, depending on the climate and your activity. You can see the need to replace that which is lost. How does this loss occur?

It occurs mainly through respiration, perspiration, urination and elimination.

Did you know you can **feel hungry** if under-hydrated? Hydration is very important in a healthy weight loss plan. Make sure you're hydrated before you reach for that snack or extra serving. If water is not a favorite beverage for you, think about adding lemon, lime, even orange or just a splash of juice or tea to the water. It's healthy and fun. You'll learn more about this subject in a few days.

How do you figure out how much you need? You will divide your body weight by two. That is the total amount of ounces of water or other clear liquid you need for the day. You'll then learn to divide that into five or six "servings" throughout the day. As soon as you wake and take care of the other necessities, you'll drink 12-20 ounces (depending on your size) of room temperature water. We suggest that you drink through a straw so that you get up to 95% water and avoid any extra air. You don't need air in your stomach.

As you enjoy other beverages throughout the day, use as much or as little ice as you prefer. If you like good cold ice water or tea, drink it with as much ice as you choose. The cold liquid will increase your metabolism.

CALCULATE YOUR WATER INTAKE

To begin, divide your body weight by two. Remember this as the amount that will replace what you lose.

Next, divide your body weight by ten. This gives you an approximate amount (in ounces) that you should consume if you divide your total into five servings per day. A 170-pound person will enjoy 17 oz. (½ liter) **five times a day.** Just drop the last number on your weight and you have 10%. (125 pounds—12-13 oz., 190 pounds—19 oz.) We suggest **no more than** 20 oz for any one beverage serving.

◆————————————————————◆

GET HEALTHY JOURNAL

Date:

"I begin each day with a glass of clean water
and stay hydrated all day."

HABIT 2: HYDRATE PROPERLY EACH DAY

My body weight = _____ Divided by 10 = _____ ounces/serving.

The times I plan on hydrating are:

I will hydrate before I snack on:

Two healthy beverages I will enjoy are:

THERE IS NO HEALTH WITHOUT HYDRATION

WEEK 1 - DAY 3

"I am learning the importance of attention to proper breathing."

HABIT 3: BREATHE EFFECTIVELY

Yesterday we mentioned that air or oxygen is the single most abundant nutrient that we take into the body. You can live up to seven weeks without food. (Extreme - but that's the average.) You can live up to seven days without water. You can live no more than seven minutes without air.

Breathing is vital to life. Proper, effective breathing is essential for metabolism and for better health. Yet, most of us are very sloppy or and lazy as it relates to our breathing ability.

If you're healthy, your lungs have the capacity of more than 15 pints of air. Because we've developed poor habits, we tend to breathe in about 3-4 pints with each breath. That obviously cheats our body of the required oxygen for normal body function. Throughout this plan you will learn a variety of ways to increase your oxygen intake. As a result you will feel better and have more energy throughout the day. For many this greatly improves their metabolism and ability to burn unwanted fat.

Begin by focusing on your ***waking breath***. As you awaken to start the new day, take about five minutes to quietly attend to getting some oxygen to the brain. The instructions for this effective activity follow in this lesson. You will also eventually find that you can do this exercise any time during the day, but it is especially beneficial before getting out of bed. Remember that our emphasis throughout this entire habit-building program is on your body's ability to revive your metabolism and energize the fat-burning mechanism.

Oxygen is fuel for your body just as food and water provide nutrients or fuel. The good news is there are no calories in oxygen. You can breathe in all you want for as long as you want and still no calories! Not only that, but the extra oxygen you take in will cause the chemical reactions in your body to take place much faster, thus, you burn more calories than you take in. This in turn speeds up your metabolism and makes you burn more fat. Oxygen is the necessary ingredient to get the fire burning for the day.

BREATHING EXERCISES

As you awaken and get ready to begin the day, take a few minutes and perform several repetitions of *5-Square breathing*. Simply **inhale** through the nose for a count of five, **hold that breath** for a count of five, **exhale** through the mouth for a count of five, and then **hold that breathless position** for the count of five.

Repeat the "5-Square" (five-five-five-five) 10 – 12 times. You have just started the "fueling" of the brain and the entire body for the day. Feel and enjoy the energy. Then get out of bed and begin the day. (Don't forget the waking water).

◆━━━━━━━━━━━━━━━━━━◆

GET HEALTHY JOURNAL

Date:

"I am learning the importance of attention to proper breathing."

HABIT 3:   BREATHE EFFECTIVELY

The most important thing I learned today is:

To improve my breathing I can:

JUMPSTART YOUR METABOLISM WITH PROPER BREATHING.

WEEK 1 - DAY 4

"I spend a few minutes each day planning my nutritional intake."

HABIT 4: PLAN TO SUCCEED

We recently attended a time management seminar. The author was asked "What is the best organizational or planning system to use"? We loved her answer. She responded, "It doesn't matter which planner you use. They all work. What matters is that you apply the system. Learn and remember ... "it works if you work it." After more than 14 years of teaching eating plans, we definitely agree. Any good eating plan will help you get where you choose to go. The key is to follow the plan one day at a time.

You have the opportunity to figure out how to personalize this planning system to help you put it to use. Each day we will continue to provide you with simple guidelines. You can write the ideas in your daily planner, keep an on-line file, or simply make sure that you have some type of journal sheet with you to note your daily activities. (Visit www.gethealthyandloseweight.com for one you can download and print.) For today, let's focus on one key planning principle. This system works because it is based on establishing the habit to: **eat every three hours.**

Obviously everyone's schedule is different, but you saw in the *Sample Eating Plan* at the beginning of the book that breakfast is listed as one hour after waking, followed by a mid-morning snack, mid-day lunch, afternoon snack, and an evening meal (at least three hours before retiring). The three-hour example that is commonly used by many people is to eat at approximately 7, 10, 1, 4, & 7.

There are few activities each day that contribute to quality of life more than your habits of eating and drinking. While it may not seem like we should have to plan these basic functions, most of the healthy people that we know, all follow a plan. It may be a worn-out cliché, but as you've heard many times: **"Failing to plan is planning to fail."** Let's **"Plan to succeed by succeeding at planning to get healthy and lose weight."**

Take a look at your schedule for the day and insert times for sensible eating. It may be four hours even five from breakfast to lunch. The variation is not a problem **when you get sufficient protein at breakfast**. The simple point is to make the time to eat 4-6 times each day. For example, plan a good time to snack in the afternoon. One of our staff orders a healthy sandwich at noon; he eats half for lunch and saves half for his afternoon snack. **Plan** your snacks and have them easily available.

PLAN TO SUCCEED

Take a few minutes today and begin to design your personal plan. Keep it simple and sensible. Who knows, this activity may help you with your overall daily planning and organization.

Think back over the last few days and ask..."When do I eat? Am I close to eating something every three hours?" Whenever we eat, we're *feeding* a habit – a habit of when we will eat and what we will eat. Create a plan to eat every three hours.

◆————————————————◆

GET HEALTHY JOURNAL

Date:

"I spend a few minutes each day planning my nutritional intake."

HABIT4: PLAN TO SUCCEED - ALWAYS

I can easily think of challenges to planning: for example, "I can't stop every three hours to eat something." I will compensate for those challenges by:

The time I will block out to do my planning is

CHOOSE THE BEST TIMES TO EAT AND DRINK.

WEEK 1 - DAY 5

"I stop what I am doing and make time to eat slowly."

HABIT 5: NOURISH WITH REAL FOOD

We have researched and gathered the principles, steps, and habits of this formula. We focused on a common-sense approach in developing these ten habits. We all agree that one principle is our favorite because it makes so much sense. That principle is: **"You are what you eat."** We've heard that in every circle. Interestingly the current popular saying in some circles at the Harvard School of Public Health is "you are what you drink."

There is obvious truth in each of these statements and yet let's take this concept a little further: **"You are what you digest or metabolize"**. You only get the benefit of the nutrients from the foods your body is able to digest and utilize. As we learn about protein, carbohydrates and lipids, you'll learn to eat the **real food** so you can get the benefit of the food enzymes. Enzymes allow the body to digest the food that you've eaten. We'll keep it simple but we'll definitely point out the benefits of this style of eating.

A while ago I (Julie) was at breakfast with my 80-year-old father. Throughout my whole life I have been a fast eater and my father was notoriously slow when eating. It had become a source of frustration for me to linger when I was finished and he had barely started. I decided to practice our own advice. I made a conscious effort to put my fork down, even counting 30 chews per bite while father slowly grazed his meal. The amazing outcomes: we finished at nearly the same time, I was not frustrated and felt comfortably full but not stuffed and bloated. I stopped rushing, chewed my food, and listened to my hunger. One of the ways to nourish ourselves is commit to stop, chew, and listen.

Stop: Remember today's commitment. "I stop what I am doing and make time to eat slowly." Train yourself to stop, chew, and listen. It is important for you to take time to eat. Sit down and focus. It's absolutely critical for a healthy lifestyle.

Chew: The most important principle of this habit is: Chew your food slowly and thoroughly. Chew your food until it is mostly liquid. You see, digestion begins in the mouth. Later we'll learn a lot more about digestion and the incredible array of food enzymes and digestive enzymes that are naturally occurring in whole foods.

Listen: If you have chosen to spend your meal time with another person, enjoy your food with some pleasant conversation. Since you are chewing, you have plenty of time to pay attention to what they are saying. If you are by yourself, pause and pay attention to your feelings and your surroundings.

TAKE TIME TO EAT

Take a few minutes today and begin to design your personal plan. Keep it simple and sensible. Who knows, this activity may help you with your overall daily planning and organization.

Think back over the last few days and ask..."When do I eat? Am I close to eating something every three hours?" Whenever we eat, we're *feeding* a habit – a habit of when we will eat and what we will eat. Create a plan to eat every three hours.

$$\blacklozenge\!\!-\!\!-\!\!-\!\!-\!\!-\!\!-\!\!-\!\!-\!\!-\!\!-\!\!-\!\!\blacklozenge$$

GET HEALTHY JOURNAL

Date:

"I stop what I am doing and make time to eat slowly."

HABIT 5: NOURISH WITH REAL FOOD

I tend to eat food too fast (when and where):

I will consume the following real foods:

I can better relax and listen while eating by:

YOU ARE WHAT YOU DIGEST.

WEEK 1 - DAY 6

"I plan some time to be active each day."

HABIT 6: MOVE TO ACTIVATE YOUR METABOLISM

Take a moment to celebrate where you are at this point. You've already moved on to Day 6. Earlier you made the commitment to learn how to eat in a healthy way. Remember you only have to take this one step at a time and continue to incorporate new ideas into your daily plan. This may be a good time to go back through your thoughts and discoveries of the week, especially review the areas where you indicated you wanted to improve.

As you saw in the Healthy Lifestyle Worksheet in the beginning of the book, there are five elements that make up our physical being. We've already discussed air (oxygen), water, and food. Today we'll consider the fourth element which is activity or motion. Tomorrow we'll practice the fifth which is rest or rejuvenation. Everything we are learning together is based on practical wisdom. It is practical, usable, and based on wisdom and the truth from the ages. There are no fads or gimmicks here. This is a way of caring for your body as we strive for a lifetime of health.

Today's commitment is to plan to be active each day. While this seems obvious, it is certainly one that is difficult for many. So let's begin to develop this habit, by forgetting most of the things we have read or heard about exercise. This is not about 30-60 minutes a day, target heart rates, or some of those seemingly foreign but impractical concepts of fitness. It is about being active in a variety of ways and in doing so, incorporating movement designed to build the body's core and to reset the all-important metabolism. We will begin to increase our strength and our daily energy. This week start being conscious and adding extra movement as a habit.

BUILD YOUR CORE STRENGTH

List all the ways in which you are normally "active" during the day. Start with walking the dog, chasing the kids, climbing flights of stairs, cleaning the house or garage, or mowing the lawn. Add to the list some other activities that get you active.

Plan some time for a walk. Make it enjoyable. Walk with a family member or a friend. Walk to the park or at the mall or someplace interesting. Your body will love you for it.

◆————————————————◆

GET HEALTHY JOURNAL

Date:

"I plan some time to be active each day."

HABIT 6: MOVE TO ACTIVATE YOUR METABOLISM

The interesting daily routine I will establish to build my core is:

The time of day I will commit to doing these activities is:

Am I keeping up with the other habits I learned? The habit that has been the most difficult for me is:

BUILD YOUR CORE BY COMMITTING TO ACTIVITY

WEEK 1 - DAY 7

Today is a break day

HABIT 7: REFRESH TO STRENGTHEN YOUR COMMITMENT

This first week is an introduction to the entire plan. You are on your way to individualizing it for your own use. You should have also made commitments to acquire some other healthy lifestyle habits.

Review your notes and results for this week. Spend some time to consider your victories. Our goal today is to have you spend time in reflection about your results, recommit to healthy habits, and to encourage you to continue on to Week 2.

◆━━━━━━━━━━━━━━━━━━━━━◆

GET HEALTHY JOURNAL

Date:

My greatest success for Week 1 was:

"IT'S NOT ENOUGH TO STARE UP THE STEPS YOU MUST STEP UP THE STAIRS."

– VANCE HAVENER

Ron & Julie Meiss

WEEK 2 - DAY 1

"I take time to plan my snacks for the day."

HABIT 1: FOCUS ON YOUR WHY

So here you are starting another week and we're back to Habit 1. That's correct. That's the design of this healthy eating course. Having worked with thousands of people we've learned that a good structure is to build the first seven of the ten habits during the first four weeks. That's what we're doing in Part I of this book. We'll then move on to the remaining three habits in Part II of this book. We'll help to strengthen your resolve to change and improve. Each time we visit Habit 1, we'll address a different issue that many people have struggled with and we'll challenge your thinking. We'll always take a moment to re-visit and remember "WHY" you've chosen to practice this course at this time.

Today's topic may appear to some of us to be so basic, and yet it is critical to our success. Remember that we've agreed to eat five times each day. At this point, one or two of our "main" meals may be smoothies or what we may choose to call blended meals. Today we'll talk about those events during mid-morning and mid-afternoon. You see, we call them snacks or mini-meals and so we often tend to not worry about them or even forget them totally.

The challenge is that these snacks are just as important to our metabolism as the other three meals. Just as kindling is used to keep a fire going when it begins to burn down, snacks help to revive our metabolism during those in-between times of the day.

Here's the key. Think about your snacks in the morning and plan them for the day. **Never** go to the vending machine or to the convenience store in hopes that you'll find just the right healthy item. Since we are constantly encouraging you to get to know Michael Pollan and his book "Food Rules", here's another of our favorites..."Never get your fuel where your car does". Finding an appropriate snack just when you need it is a difficult task for the most talented seeker. Have your snacks available for the day, and set up a reminder when it's time. We are committed to eating every three hours. Appropriate snacks help us fill the nutritional gap and keep us going.

PLAN YOUR SNACKS

Make a list of your favorite snacks. Brainstorm with a friend who knows your eating habits to come up with creative healthy snacks. At *www.gethealthyandloseweight.com*, there is a guide to healthy snacks and smoothies under *Resources* Remember as you are planning and enjoying your snacks, while it may be just a 200-calorie meal bar, it is a mini-meal. Slow down and enjoy it.

———◆———

GET HEALTHY JOURNAL

Date:

"I take time to plan my snacks for the day."

HABIT 1: FOCUS ON YOUR WHY

On Week 1 Day 1 you learned to focus on your reason to achieve a healthy weight. This is a good time reflect and review your thinking. What additional thoughts have you had?

How has your thinking changed?

How fit and healthy do you want to be at age 75?

GET SERIOUS ABOUT GETTING HEALTHY

WEEK 2 - DAY 2

"I am careful to reduce my intake of sweetened beverages."

HABIT 2: HYDRATE PROPERLY

Take time for a quick review of your water intake. We're now striving to consume about half our body weight in ounces of water each day. Of course, every serving of tea or lightly flavored water counts toward that total and even eating fruits and vegetables in their "live" state contributes to your water needs. Soup, milk, unsweetened tea and those tasty blended meals (smoothies) that you might want to enjoy each day, also hydrate the body and add to the total.

Interestingly, some of the "common" beverages do not count. Coffee, cola, and beer do not help to hydrate the body because they tend to act as a diuretic, flushing water from the body. Some of our doctor friends advise that for every cup of coffee or other caffeinated drink, you need to add that many ounces to your daily water total. We are not saying that you should not drink coffee, but we do want you to know that it does not contribute to your water totals for the day.

We doubt that this will come as a surprise to you at this time, but it is time to recommend that you move toward eliminating all of the sweetened beverages available in the store cooler. We'll learn much more about the dangers of added sugar (especially "weird stuff" like high fructose corn syrup) in our beverages later on.

For now, it is best to replace those sweetened beverages with water, lightly-flavored water, unsweetened tea, or some of the newer offerings that use natural sweeteners. The main problem is this.... the majority of the sweeteners used in beverages today are forms of high fructose corn syrup. This un-natural concoction does not break down in the body in the same way as regular sugar (sucrose) and is a likely contributor to many of our health problems today.

Carefully journal your beverage intake for a few days and discuss with a partner. If it is helpful, use the food diary sheet available at the Get Healthy and Lose Weight website. Watch the calorie content of your beverages. Make a commitment that you will not drink your calories in sweetened beverages.

WATCH YOUR BEVERAGE INTAKE

Find a beverage container that is easy for you to use and has about the right number of ounces, i.e. a 16 ounce reusable water bottle, a 20 or 24 ounce reusable cup with reusable straw. Then you simply have to fill it 5 or 6 times in a day and you have taken in all your beverages.

Another hint is set out your waking water the night before, you can actually drink more room temperature water and you won't forget it. Try by the coffee pot or even by the bathroom sink so you see it first thing on waking. A final hint, don't forget the Week 1 - Day 2 suggestion that you drink through a straw.

✦━━━━━━━━━━━━━━━━━━━━━━━━━✦

GET HEALTHY JOURNAL

Date:

"I am careful to reduce my intake of sweetened beverages."

HABIT 2: HYDRATE PROPERLY

How committed have I been to drinking the right amount of water (Week 1 – Day 2) on a daily basis?

What substitute beverages am I learning to use for sweetened beverages?

PROPER HYDRATION IS VITAL

WEEK 2 - DAY 3

"I will take time each day to practice power breathing."

HABIT 3: BREATHE EFFECTIVELY

Just think how good you might feel if you took a few minutes each day and did 5-Square breathing. You are waking that way most mornings, right? Take 5 minutes in the morning and get some oxygen to the brain. After all, we've been hibernating all night ... we need to wake up! We have conducted 90-day weight loss sessions that were focused exclusively on breathing, and some participants experienced dramatic weight loss. You may want to get a copy of the book, *Jumpstart Your Metabolism: How To Lose Weight By Changing The Way You Breathe*, by Pam Grout. It's filled with many great exercises.

Chopping Wood ... today we'll take the time to learn an excellent form of **power breathing** that you can practice two or three times during the day. This exercise, which is often called, *Chopping Wood*, is an excellent way to drive stale air out of the lower lung area and make room for fresh aerobic energy. It is a practical way to increase your oxygen uptake throughout the day. Here's how you do it:

1. Stand with your feet shoulder width apart, arms stretched in front of you with fingers clasped.

2. As you inhale through the nose raise your arms slowly above your head. Hold for a count of 5.

3. Exhale forcefully as you drop your arms to the floor as if chopping wood. Bend your knees slightly and continue the motion through your open legs and hold for a count of 5.

4. Inhale slowly as you return to the position of your arms above your head. Continue for 10 repetitions.

START *CHOPPING*

Chopping Wood is a great activity to practice late morning and/or late afternoon. Taking just a couple of minutes before eating your main meals of the day, will not only revitalize you at the time, but along with a glass of water, will help curb your hunger as you sit down to eat. Wear comfortable clothing as always when you are engaging any form of activity.

This exercise that we are comparing to wood-chopping is an example of an activity that is totally new and requires us to learn a completely new habit.

◆——————————————◆

GET HEALTHY JOURNAL

Date:

"I take time each day to practice power breathing."

HABIT 3: BREATHE EFFECTIVELY

How will I remind myself to incorporate this activity into my daily routine most days?

What are other similar breathing exercises that I have performed at other times in my life that I may choose to start again?

FILL YOUR LUNGS WITH ENERGY WITH EACH BREATH

Week 2 - Day 4

"I do 'what it takes' to stick to my eating plan each day."

HABIT 4: PLAN TO SUCCEED

Let's take a close look at the entire day as it relates to your new habits of eating and drinking. We know that we enjoy a water during the first hour after waking. Remember that it is the number of ounces equal to 10% of your body weight. That water is followed by a healthy breakfast about one hour after waking. Whether you are enjoying a blended shake for breakfast or having something else, this is the **most important** meal of the day. You are ending a 12 hour fast.

It's now clear that our goal is to eat every three hours, five times a day, meaning that our last meal is 12 hours after the first meal. The meal timing is probably starting to make sense by now, but how about the timing of your beverages? Perhaps this guideline will help: **eat five times a day - have 5 beverages between meal times**

That statement may simplify things and help make sense for your planning. The day consists of three meals and two snacks (mini-meals) spaced as close to three hours apart as your schedule allows. Additionally there are 5 beverages in between the meal times. Later you will learn why you should not consume beverages with your meals.

Why do we recommend 5 small meals per day for people that are finally trying to get control over their eating habits? A lot of us who are used to eating two to three meals per day easily can **eat way too many calories in one sitting.** By eating smaller meals every three hours throughout the day, it helps to get control over the amount that you eat.

Think about this "day in the life" of the average person at the office – you eat lunch at noon, and then don't eat dinner until getting home at about 7:00 pm that night. You were so busy at work that you forgot to eat any mini-meal or snack mid-afternoon. With six to seven hours between meals, you're so ravenous when you get home that you **"inhale"** 2,000 calories before you've even given your brain a chance to register that you've eaten this much. The end result: eating **way more** in a day than your body can burn for energy.

EVALUATE YOUR PLAN

You've been planning your nourishment and hydration for about 10 days. Do a quick review to see what is making sense and working for you. As you are learning, when we build a firm foundation of eating and drinking habits, there are a number of finishing touches that really help to build a strong plan.

Do you have a helpful planning tip? Visit the blog at the Get Healthy and Lose Weight Website to share it with others.

◆————————————————————◆

GET HEALTHY JOURNAL

Date:

I do 'what it takes' to stick to my eating plan each day."

HABIT 4: CREATE A PERSONAL, DAILY PLAN

What is something that I continue to struggle with?

What is one thing I have learned about planning my eating and drinking schedule that has helped me already?

FAST FOR 12 HOURS ... THEN 5 MEALS AND 5 BEVERAGES

WEEK 2 - DAY 5

"I realize the importance of eating high-quality protein."

HABIT 5: NOURISH WITH REAL FOOD

You've probably wondered how we have gone almost two weeks without spending a lot of time focusing on what and on how much we should eat and drink. For now we still want to keep it simple. There's not that much to learn about the actual food types and food groups while we are focusing on developing the healthy habits.

The good news is that there are only three types of food. This is not to be confused with the fact that there are a number of food groups and there are certainly many choices. The manager of our local supermarket told us recently that there are more than 50,000 different items in her store to choose from. You can easily see why we're going to focus on just the three food types.

Everything that we eat is in the form of: **proteins, carbohydrates or lipids**. Lipids are commonly referred to as fats and they are actually both fats and oils. We have a full week of lessons on these important foods. For the moment, we are creating the balance of these three types by helping with your meal timing and other important factors such as eliminating some of the harmful "food-like substances".

Carbohydrates are all of the foods that contain carbon, oxygen and hydrogen. You can plainly see that is where the name comes from. Once again, Week 6 of this healthy eating plan will introduce us to the fruits, vegetables, grains and other food groups that are included in this important food type.

As we continue to learn healthy habits, you will discover much more about each of these food categories. You will find, for instance, that a typical day is made up of a total intake of about 50% carbohydrate, 25% protein, and 25% lipids. As we continue to learn to healthy eating habits, the percentages, serving sizes and even the number of calories will all make sense and will be easier to understand.

Protein will covered in detail when we get to Week 5. If you are beginning to sense that you would like to know more about food at this time, please feel free to turn to that section and begin to understand more about protein. You will learn that there are both animal and plant sources of protein.

A very effective way of insuring adequate protein each day is to enjoy healthy and tasty protein smoothies or shakes. Perhaps the best example of using protein in a powdered form is to begin each day with what we often call a "blended" meal which combines a form of protein with valuable fruits and nuts, providing an excellent way to break the fast. There are clearly some important tips to learn about creating healthy protein-based smoothies.

EAT HEALTHY PROTEINS

Learn to get creative with your protein meal replacements. What is the right amount of protein per serving? The answer is about 15 grams which is the equivalent of 2 ounces of chicken or a similar protein source. Remember to take time to slow down and enjoy the "smoothie". Be sure and try the suggestions that use plain yogurt as the base. You may enjoy the "thickness".

◆————————————————————◆

GET HEALTHY JOURNAL

Date:

"I realize the importance of eating high-quality protein."

HABIT 5: NOURISH WITH REAL FOOD

What is something that I continue to struggle with?

What is one thing I have learned about planning my eating and drinking schedule that has helped me thus far?

PROTEIN MEANS A "HEALTHY PROTEIN."

WEEK 2 - DAY 6

"I build my core to build my strength."

HABIT 6: MOVE TO ACTIVATE YOUR METABOLISM

It's time again to focus on movement to strengthen our core. Our balanced protein intake each day is helping us build lean muscle tissue which should create an increase in metabolism. **When we build lean muscle it helps us burn fat.** The activities that we learn here will help us build a strong core to support the muscle strength.

With that in mind, today is all about some additional activities to build your core strength. Start slow with about five repetitions and gradually build up to 21. Let's learn three core builders:

1. Build Balance: stand comfortably, arms outstretched to the side with palms down, look straight ahead and begin to turn slowly clockwise then rotate counter clockwise. Complete one or two rotations and then stop to make sure you are not getting dizzy. Complete five rotations slowly. Gradually work up to 21 rotations.

2. Lie comfortably on a soft floor, mat, or rug. With your arms at your side, palms down, slowly raise your legs bringing them up

straight above the hips. Slowly lower your legs back to the floor. Begin with 5 repetitions. You will gradually work up to 21 lifts.

3. Move to a kneeling position with your arms at your side. Slowly move your shoulders back and slightly arch your back. Go a short distance but do not strain and then return. It strengthens your back and stomach core muscles. Begin with 5 and slowly work your way to 21 repetitions.

These are the first three of five motions that you will come to know as the "master motions". Again, we realize that this type of activity may be very new to you and will require some discipline to build into your daily activities. It's fine to do it gradually (progress, not perfection), and to insure that this healthy weight system works for you, each activity and each habit is very important.

CHOP WOOD AND BUILD YOUR CORE

Make sure to take time to *Chop Wood* once or twice a day (See: Week 2 – Day 3). It's great for stretching and breathing. Set aside about 10 minutes once or twice a day, to Chop Wood and practice the three core builders that we just demonstrated. Continue to find additional ways to be active and build your core each day. Walking is still our favorite.

◆———————————————————◆

GET HEALTHY JOURNAL

Date:

"I build my core to build my strength."

HABIT 6: MOVE TO ACTIVATE YOUR METABOLISM

One thing I learned today is:

My first (honest) reaction to the Master Motions is:

One thing I am especially committed to working on is

BUILD LEAN MUSCLE TO BURN FAT

Week 2 - Day 7

Today is a break day

HABIT 7: REFRESH TO STRENGTHEN YOUR COMMITMENT

A lifestyle coach recently said, "This is not a plan for the people who need it and it really isn't just a plan for the people who want it; It's a plan **for the people who do it.**" Your new habits cannot be learned by reading a book, getting a CD or DVD. You get them by **practicing them on a daily basis**. They become your daily routine when you **do them over and over** until they become lifestyle habits. John Maxwell says, "Forget motivation. Just do it. Exercise, lose weight, test your blood sugar, or whatever. Do it without motivation. And then, guess what? After you start doing the thing, that's when the motivation comes" and makes it easy for you to keep on doing it.

◆———————————————————◆

GET HEALTHY JOURNAL

Date:

The habits I practiced daily during Week 2 are:

"JUST DO IT"

WEEK 3 - DAY 1

"Sharing this plan with others helps me learn more about it."

HABIT 1: FOCUS ON YOUR "WHY"

We have now been researching, learning, and sharing these nutrition guidelines with others for more than 15 years. While we have continued to learn, one thing has become obvious. The basic principles of healthy eating do not change. Fads may come and go; practical wisdom is timeless. You've probably already discovered that **we all gain in our commitment and growth when we share our successes and errors with the people around us**. Think of people who are with you on a regular basis and/or people who really care about you and how you are doing. It's time to start telling them about your health pursuits and how this is working for you.

Here is one of our favorites. Diane P. came to us in September, 1998. Her husband of nearly 30 years had just won a cruise experience for the two of them, and she had 6 weeks to lose 16 pounds. Diane was so committed to this goal that we soon realized that there was no way she would allow herself to fail. She ate every 3 hours, drank her water 5 times a day, went for a walk with her husband every evening when he got home, and looked and felt great on that November cruise. We know because we got to see the pictures. Diane's "Why" was so strong that she thought about it every day and shared it with anyone who would listen.

Re-visit your "Why" worksheet at the beginning of the book. Did you list the reasons that are really important to you? Take some time and really think this through. It must be a personal, emotional reason for making the commitment.

Another favorite "Why" we've heard was from a woman who said that money was tight for her family at the time that she was getting healthy and losing weight, and she really looked forward to being able to "go shopping in the back part of her closet". Do you have any great clothes that just don't fit anymore?

Your "Why" may be a health reason; in our experience it usually is. It may be how your clothes feel or look; more than likely, it may involve how you feel - the amount of energy that is less than you used to have. Ask yourself some serious questions about your health. Are there any health concerns that you haven't addressed? Are there some tests that you've put off because you're not sure you really want to know what the outcome might be. Whatever your "WHY", this would be a good time to internalize it, and then go out and share it with others. It will help you succeed in staying on task and accomplishing your goals.

REVISIT YOUR "WHY"

You've undoubtedly heard the saying that we can endure any "How" if our "Why" is strong enough. Make sure your goal is clear. Spend time this week and re-visit your commitment.

Pick at least one of your favorite ideas from this program. Maybe it's getting some breakfast each morning, or eating every 3 hours so you don't get hungry. Pick something that you like and find time to share those thoughts with others.

◆────────────────────────◆

GET HEALTHY JOURNAL

Date :

"Sharing this plan with others helps me learn more about it."

HABIT 1: FOCUS ON YOUR "WHY"

Who are the people that I can think of to share all my ideas with?

What will I talk about for starters?

What is one way I can best share my ideas?

IF YOU REALLY CARE......SHARE

WEEK 3 - DAY 2

"I avoid the pitfalls of artificial sweeteners."

Habit 2: HYDRATE PROPERLY

The authors of the current Harvard School of Public Health eating program have written that "we are what we drink." It was one week ago that we learned we should not get our calories in our beverages. Many authors in this field strongly suggest that we do not have an eating problem, but rather we have a drinking problem. Of course, most researchers are finding that we really have both. It may seem that the answer to not drinking calories would be to turn to diet drinks, but you've undoubtedly heard that artificial sweeteners seem to do more to make us fat rather than to help us. We have several books and reports we can recommend on the subject at our website that support this concept and other reports we can refer you to. Please contact us.

Avoid all forms of artificial sweeteners. Your eating goal is to put natural foods into your body, not artificial, non-nutritive, chemically-produced products. These include:

1. Saccharin (Sweet'n Low, Sugar Twin, Sucaryl),

2. Sucralose (Splenda)

3. Aspartame (Equal, NutraSweet)

4. Acesulfame potassium (Sunette, Sweet One)

These are the culprits and are commonly found in sodas, teas, water, and other artificially sweetened beverages. One exception is Stevia – considered to be healthy and a useful sweetener. **Artificial sweeteners of all types are chemically produced, non-nutritive sugar substitutes**. Truly the best choice when choosing an artificial sweetener is none of the above with the exception of Stevia. There are health concerns with non-nutritive sweeteners because they are **all unnatural and chemically produced**. Each artificial sweetener has its own problems and it is doubtful that this type of substance can help us reach our goal of healthy weight.

Let's get personal and a bit more serious before we leave this thought. If diet sodas and other artificially-sweetened beverages helped to make us healthier, most of us would look and feel a lot better. If you still doubt this, cut back and then totally eliminate these types of drinks for a couple of weeks. It is our experience that you will gradually feel a lot more energy from drinkinging cleaner beverages, and you will not have any desire to go back. You've come this far. Aren't you ready for another major step toward optimal health?

RESEARCH IT FOR YOURSELF

Take some time and do some research for yourself. There just does not seem to be any healthy reason to consume these un-natural substances. At least cut back for now, and be very careful about offering these artificial question marks to your children or anyone else you love. Instead, continue to seek ways to enjoy "flavored" water, teas, and safer, healthier beverages.

◆————————————————◆

GET HEALTHY JOURNAL

Date:

"I avoid the pitfalls of artificial sweeteners."

HABIT 2: HYDRATE PROPERLY

What is one thing I can do to improve on the quality of the beverages that I use to hydrate?

What is one thing I am really committed to working on?

THE COLORED PACKETS ARE CALLED "ARTIFICIAL" FOR A REASON

WEEK 3 - DAY 3

"I am learning variations of power breathing."

HABIT 3: BREATHE EFFECTIVELY

You've undoubtedly noticed that it is very easy to use the analogy of a fire when we are speaking of metabolism. You know a fire cannot burn without oxygen. Today think about the fact that the process of metabolism cannot take place in the body without sufficient oxygen. Earlier we reflected on the fact that just a few minutes without oxygen and life will be extinguished. Likewise, without sufficient oxygen our body cannot burn the nutrients that we consume.

Begin each day with a few minutes of basic 5-Square breathing covered in Week 1 – Day 3. Then, take a break once or twice a day and Chop Wood (Week 2 – Day 3). Enhance your Chop Wood exercise by holding the upper and the lower position for a count of five. In other words, raise your arms over your head, stretch and hold for a count of 5. When you reach a position with your arms between your legs and complete exhalation, hold for a count of 5. It is the hold position that assists your body with fat burning.

When you find yourself with a minute or two of "wait" time during the day, practice some 5-Square breathing with this "twist". When you inhale, allow the breath to go deep into your lungs and feel your stomach (actually the diaphragm) begin to expand rather than puffing up your chest. If possible, lie flat for a few minutes and practice this exercise. When lying on your back you will find it easier to perform this natural breathing movement. Place one hand comfortably on your stomach and feel it rise as you inhale. Remember that we always inhale gently through the nose, and exhale forcefully and completely through the mouth with our lips puckered.

It seems as though this week is becoming a true reality check, so please allow us another personal moment here. We've worked with thousands of people and have learned that this (breathing) information is often the most difficult new idea to incorporate. It appears that because breathing is an autonomic response (we do it without thinking), it requires a thoughtful effort to spend some time thinking about it and learning to practice these exercises. Ironically, this is also the one habit that stands the greatest chance of providing a breakthrough for you on your journey to regaining your health.

We strongly encourage you to give this breathing stuff some time and energy. As the habit suggests, it is time to learn to breathe effectively.

THE POWER OF PROPER BREATHING

As you take time to perform 5-Square breathing, notice how much better you feel as the oxygen makes its way to your brain. Imagine the other life-giving benefits.

Talk to a singer you know and ask them to teach you something about proper breathing. Great vocalists and public speakers have mastered the power of proper breathing.

———◆————————————————◆———

GET HEALTHY JOURNAL

Date:

"I learn variations of power breathing."

HABIT 3: BREATHE EFFECTIVELY

How do I feel that I am doing on the job of proper breathing?

What is something I need to pay more attention to?

TAKE TIME TODAY FOR "A BREATH OF FRESH AIR"

Week 3 - Day 4

"I will always find creative ways to set up reminders."

HABIT 4: PLAN TO SUCCEED

We continue now with our numbers discussion for this week. We've spent some time reinforcing the importance of learning to eat every three hours. We quickly realized that meant that we would eat at least five times each day and have a healthy beverage five times each day. We've also learning not to combine the eating and the drinking.

Let's focus on another number. The number is 12. One of our favorite eating courses begins with "the principle of the 12 and 12". Here's the concept: **Our life must fit into a 24-hour day.** We've probably felt that there aren't enough hours in the day, that we never have enough time, or maybe, it just seems we don't have as much time as we used to. Silly, isn't it? While we all know what we mean when saying those things, the truth is that we all have the same number of seconds, minutes, and hours, in each day. We learn to fit into those 24 hour time frames. The fact is that we really don't manage time. Rather, we manage our activities and our interactions within the allotted time. This is a very helpful mindset to realize.

The principle of 12 and 12 is based on the fact that our bodies seem to work best in today's busy lifestyle when we learn to **fast for 12 and then burn for 12**. You may not have thought of it that way, but we do well when we fast (no eating and drinking) for 12 hours. For the average person that would likely be from 7 p.m. To 7 a.m. Then we eat, drink, and move (burn) for 12 hours. Using the above example we would then resume eating and drinking around 7 a.m. This means that we learn to fit the 3-hour rule (eat every 3 hours) and fit the 5 and 5 (eat 5 times each day and drink 5 beverages each day) between the hours of 7 and 7 during the day. Again, you may need to adjust your schedule but the principle is the same.

This seems like a good time to reinforce a principle that we'll state several times in a variety of ways. This is not about being perfect. This is about learning the principles and then applying them on a daily basis in the best way that we are able. The number here to keep in mind is 80-20. Strive to be on target at least 80% of the time. You know this concept. Success can be achieved when we learn to practice these principle most of the time. We have learned from experience that a very realistic goal is 80%.

Is that too many numbers for you? As we learn to plan and to keep score, it helps to know the rules and the boundaries. So, now we know.

IMPROVE YOUR PLANNING

This is an appropriate time to improve your planning. Set up reminders so that even when you're busy, you get your snack, your lunch, and your important beverages.

Figure better ways to invest your time. Get back to using a planner or set up a calendar on your computer. Put an app on your phone or subscribe to a text service that will help with reminders.

◆————————————————◆

GET HEALTHY JOURNAL

Date :

"I will always find creative ways to set up reminders."

HABIT 4: PLAN TO SUCCEED

What will I do to improve my planning?

What have I succeeded at in my previous planning efforts?

LEARN WAYS TO "INVEST YOUR TIME WISELY"

WEEK 3 - DAY 5

"I will choose to eat healthy carbs."

HABIT 5: NOURISH WITH REAL FOOD

Last week we talked about one of the foods types that we know as protein. Protein means of first quality and it is the building material of the body and most of its components. Look at yourself: skin, hair, nails ... all protein. Even the hormones that we talk about in a program like this are composed of protein. We are learning the many ways that we can feed our body healthy protein.

Today we introduce the second food type, which is undoubtedly the most misunderstood. That is carbohydrates. A carbohydrate is a combination of carbon, oxygen and hydrogen. Carbohydrates make up the largest of the food types, and are found primarily in fruit, vegetable, grain and fiber. Starchy vegetables such as corn and potatoes are carbohydrates.

What carbohydrates should you eat and how much? Let's look at some guidelines to start out with:

- **Vegetables:** eat all you will. You will learn to limit potatoes and corn as they act like starches.

- **Fruit:** eat small servings and always limit fruit juice to 4 ounces.

- **Grains:** eat only whole grains (go light on white) and enjoy 2 servings per day. Fiber: add fiber to your breakfast.

Here are some key definition that we will use:

Whole foods. They are foods that are unprocessed and unrefined, or processed and refined as little as possible before being consumed. Whole foods typically do not contain added ingredients, such as sugar, salt, or fat. Examples of whole foods include fruits and vegetables, unprocessed meat, poultry, and fish, and non-homogenized milk. The term is often confused with organic food, but whole foods are not necessarily organic, nor are organic foods necessarily whole. There are several ways to meet the body's needs with respect to whole foods. One way is to consume a variety of fresh raw fruits, vegetables and whole grains every day. The following definitions will help clarity the difference.

Real foods. Real foods contains all of the nutrients that are necessary for the body to assimilate and utilize for maintenance and health, and will not "cost" the body to put to use.

Processed foods. Process foods are often called junk foods. Processed food is a substance that is missing some of the nutrients that the body requires for health, and will cost energy and other nutrients to put to use. For now, add as much fresh vegetable as you can to the meal that you are enjoying each day. There are so many wonderful raw foods that will help you meet all of your carbohydrate goals. As we are known to say repeatedly…"Your body will love you".

EAT THE RIGHT CARBS

Eat your veggies. Choose colorful vegetables other than potatoes or corn. Stay away from fruit juice for now. Without the fiber, it's awfully high in sugar. There's a reason that a juice glass is only 4 ounces. Whole fresh fruit is a better choice.

◆——————————————————◆

GET HEALTHY JOURNAL

Date:

"I will choose to eat healthy carbs."

HABIT 5: NOURISH WITH REAL FOOD

What vegetables do I plan to enjoy?

What other carbs will I eat?

How can I learn to incorporate more raw food into my diet?

EAT ALL OF THE COLORS OF THE RAINBOW

Week 3 - Day 6

"I take time to strengthen my body each day."

HABIT 6: MOVE TO ACTIVATE YOUR METABOLISM

We started learning to move with a series of movements that have been used for thousands of years. Go back to Week 2 – Day 6 and review the movements you have learned so far. Practice each of these daily as you continue to build up to 21 repetitions. Today we will add two more which are important strength builders, practiced with the sole intent of building and strengthening your body's core.

As you perform the first three of the **Master Motions** (rotate, leg lift, back arch) which we learned earlier, continue on with **this new motion as the fourth:**

1. Begin seated comfortably on the floor with your arms at your side, palms resting on the floor.

2. Slowly raise your torso, drop your head back, and move up to a position of your midsection becoming parallel with the floor. Your lower legs, midsection, and your arms will come to be in the shape of a table.

3. Slowly return to a seated position.

Repeat this motion several times and gradually add repetitions until you reach a total of 21.

Here is the fifth in the Master Motions:

1. Kneel and slowly lean forward to a "pushup" position with your palms and your knees comfortably supporting your body.

2. Slowly raise your midsection to a high, arched position (buttocks highest) and hold.

3. Slowly lower the midsection, knees remaining off the floor, and body gently sagging (slight U position).

Rise up to the heightened position and repeat motion several times. Do not strain. Your goal is to improve to 21 repetitions. **Do not attempt these motions if you have any back, shoulder, or other joint problems.** Start slowly and always consult a physician or other medical professional before beginning these (or any) exercises of this type.

This series of motions has proven extremely beneficial to thousands of participants over the past 14 years. We recommend that you check www.gethealthyandloseweight.com for alternative exercises.

PUTTING IT TOGETHER

Here is a tip about how to use the Master Motions. Begin by Chopping Wood. Then perform each of these 5 exercises, gradually working your way up to 21 repetitions of each. There is a detailed instruction guide on our website.

◆————————————————————————◆

GET HEALTHY JOURNAL

Date:

"I take time to strengthen my body each day."

HABIT 6: MOVE TO ACTIVATE YOUR METABOLISM

Have I been moving? How many repetitions have I worked up to of the first three Master Motions?

How many repetitions of the fourth and fifth Master Motions do I think I should start with?

LEARN THE MASTER MOTIONS

WEEK 3 - DAY 7

Today is a break day

HABIT 7: REFRESH TO STRENGTHEN YOUR COMMITMENT

We know from many years of experience that taking a day off each week is very important to the success of this program. In fact, if you're in the middle of a crazy day and you realize that you may not get to your activities for the day, give yourself permission to skip a day. Remember:. Strive to be on target at least 80% of the time.

◆————————————————◆

GET HEALTHY JOURNAL

Date:

Think back to Week 1 – Day 1. What do you think has been your greatest accomplishment?

NOTHING TASTES AS GOOD AS HEALTHY WEIGHT FEELS

Ron & Julie Meiss

WEEK 4 - DAY 1

"As I see improvement in my health,

I choose to keep learning."

HABIT 1: FOCUS ON YOUR WHY

The popular belief about changing behavior has typically stated that "it takes 21 days to permanently alter the way you do things". That came as the result of some studies conducted in the late 1940s. Additional research in the past 10 years by the world's largest weight loss organization, suggests that the time required for permanent change is much closer to 40 days, and perhaps even longer depending on the complexity of the behavior. That's a somewhat complicated way of saying that as we begin week four together, we are making progress and are probably more than half way to creating new habits that will last a lifetime. The name of today's habit was chosen for a reason. We must continue to remember the Why.

Think of all the things we've learned together. How much better do you feel than you did last month at this time? Do some of your clothes fit better? Has your energy level improved?

Since you're answering in the positive, it is a good time to continue looking forward. Spend a few minutes now and review your objectives and progress. Remember, you are learning to eat in a way that will create a lifetime of health.

We suggest that you learn to work on one aspect at a time. Some of us have been learning and practicing these concepts for several years now, and it is still rewarding to realize we are continuing to make small improvements. For example, have you learned to make sure that you get your breakfast about one hour after waking? There are a number of reasons that we wake up with a "waking breath" exercise, enjoy our first water of the day, and then follow with breakfast. Remember, break-the-fast. Get your metabolism working.

Here's another reminder from two weeks ago. The mid-morning and the mid-afternoon snack or mini-meal is a very important step. It is also the habit that is the easiest to forget. Plan your snacks for the day. Do not leave any room to fail. The last thing you want is to be standing at the vending machine or looking at the junk at the convenience store to help "tide you over". Remember that you have the power of choice. At this point in your life you realize that the people who get what they want out of life do not just have a great day. They do what it takes to "make it a great day".

RECOMMIT

Recommit to the habits you learned earlier and decide what your next steps will be as you continue to learn to eat healthy. Pick a favorite breakfast from what we have learned to this point. Enjoy it tomorrow and recommit to making breakfast the most important meal of the day.

◆———————————————◆

GET HEALTHY JOURNAL

Date:

"As I can see improvement in my health,

I choose to keep learning."

HABIT 1: FOCUS ON YOUR WHY

What is one thing that has become clear to me over the past three weeks?"

What area do I know that I need to recommit to?

OUR GOAL IS PROGRESS RATHER THAN PERFECTION

Week 4 - Day 2

"I make sure that I enjoy my favorite drinks throughout the day."

HABIT 2: HYDRATE PROPERLY

We recently compared the information that we are sharing now, with similar plans that were written 10-12 years ago. By far, the most significant changes are in the lessons that have to do with hydration. As we've learned, sweeteners and artificial sweeteners have dramatically changed the beverage market. We recently overheard a customer at a large convenience store remark, "There's not one beverage in that entire cooler that's fit to drink". That may be a bit of an exaggeration, but it certainly is close to the truth.

Careful attention to your beverage intake has had a lot to do with your success this past month. You've noticed that we emphasize the value of enjoying a full beverage about 30 minutes before a meal. It helps with the feeling of feeling full and satisfied.

Another hydration principle has been mentioned, but not fully explained. It is important to enjoy your beverages between meal times and not with your meals. For example, have your waking beverage during the first hour of your day, and then enjoy breakfast. Even a small glass of fruit juice is better served just before your meal. If you find this difficult at first, have a glass of room temperature water on the table while you eat, but not a beverage containing ice.

There are several factors involved here. Perhaps the most important is the fact that we tend to eat faster when we wash down our food with a drink. There are also studies that suggest that consuming a lot of liquid while eating dilutes the digestive fluids and hampers the body's ability to break down the food. One thing is for certain. While the digestion process is taking place, it makes no sense to pour iced beverage into the area where the food is being prepared for the process of metabolism. In a sense, pouring the iced drink right into the mix is actually putting out the fire. We know for sure that ice water definitely interferes with the digestion of lipids. Save the ice cold beverage for later. Allow the digestion process to take place. Avoid some of the gassy, bloated feeling after eating that you had come to believe was normal.

One other key reminder about your daily intake of fluids. It is possible to consume 5-10 ounces of liquid each day from the food that you eat. In Week 6 we will learn a great deal about the carbohydrates that we know as fruits and vegetables. You will discover that when consumed raw or live, these colorful foods are filled with hundreds of healthy nutrients AND much of it is in the form of liquid. The key is to remember that we are talking about eating the actual food and not just the juice. Although juicing can be very healthy, it is important to eat the entire plant to benefit from all of the nutrients.

ENJOY YOUR BEVERAGES

Enjoy a beverage before your meal. Then take time to chew your food thoroughly until it becomes liquid. Continue to try different teas and other healthy drinks. Many bottled beverages are being improved, but for now many are not fit to drink.

◆———————————————————◆

GET HEALTHY JOURNAL

Date:

"I make sure that I enjoy my favorite drinks throughout the day."

HABIT 2: HYDRATE PROPERLY

What was the most interesting thing I learned today?

How many ounces of fluid am I now consuming during each of the five intervals per day?

I ENJOY 10% OF MY BODY WEIGHT

IN OUNCES OF FLUID FIVE TIMES PER DAY

WEEK 4 - DAY 3

"I will continue to increase my activity and my lungpower."

HABIT 3: BREATHE EFFECTIVELY

This important habit reminds us of the importance of taking in sufficient oxygen throughout the day to sustain metabolism and muscle growth, both of which are vital to getting healthy. You have also undoubtedly noticed that there is a wonderful connection between breathing and the strength-building activities that we learn on Day 6. Let's take a closer look at the relationship between learning to breathe effectively and keeping yourself active.

We discovered at the very beginning of our research that there are a number of misconceptions about what is involved in order to create the many benefits of exercise. A major fitness organization recently surveyed potential clients. Nearly 100% indicated that they were sure that they needed more activity, and only about 30% said that they were committed to doing so. The two main reasons given for not being willing were: "not enough time" and "it's just too hard".

For most of us, time is an issue. That's the main reason that we have been suggesting activities that can be fit into a busy day and do not require driving somewhere or having special clothing. You have learned to chop wood, practice 5-Square breathing, and perform the Master Motions that help strengthen the body's core.

You have learned to look for ways to increase the amount of steps you take, for example, after parking your car or doing your daily shopping. The good news is that we know today that it all counts. Fitness is not just what takes place at a fitness center or an aerobics studio. It is about the total amount of activity that we get in a day.

Effective breathing is absolutely critical to the success of any purposeful activity. Even while sitting as you are on hold or waiting for some function to take place on your computer, you can fit in a few squares of breathing.

This is not to say that all of the things that you've been told over the past years have been wrong. When aerobics came on the scene more than 40 years ago, it seemed like the answer. It is not the only answer.

What we've done so far is part of preparing your mind and your body to be ready for some powerful information that will help "get you into shape" quickly and easily. There is no equipment or clothing that you need to buy. You will continue to learn effective methods to increase your daily activity and your lungpower. Keep improving your breathing and building up your lung power. Day 6 this week will be the beginning of a whole new way of looking at keeping the body active.

HOW IS YOUR BREATHING?

Take a couple of minutes today and jot down your perceptions about breathing and exercise. Where did you learn these perceptions? Be willing to keep an open mind.

Where are you now? Rate yourself on a scale of 1 to 5 with 1 indicating that you are in excellent shape and you know what it takes to stay there. On the other end of the spectrum, 5 is an admission that you are out of shape.

$\blacklozenge$ ——————————————————— $\blacklozenge$

GET HEALTHY JOURNAL

Date:

"I will continue to increase my activity and my lungpower."

HABIT 3: BREATHE EFFECTIVELY

What relationship do my breathing activities have with the five Master Motions?

How often do I take the time to perform the suggested breathing activities before doing the Master Motions?

OXYGEN KEEPS THE FIRE BURNING

WEEK 4 - DAY 4

"I maintain a healthy balance of the three food types."

HABIT 4: PLAN TO SUCCEED

You have to first plan this nutrition journey; then you create a planning process that can be used on a daily basis to keep you on track. That's why you would weigh yourself; that's why you might measure from time to time, or try on different pieces of clothing. It allows you to keep score - to know what your current status is. Another thought about knowing where you stand ... A friend went to a major university during the 1960s and the school did away with the grading process. Everyone got a grade of pass or fail. Our friend went crazy. She didn't know how she was doing. She had no way of keeping score.

It's certainly possible to spend too much time and energy keeping score, but there is at least one more set of numbers that you will benefit from knowing as we progress to some new habits. The new score you will learn is the ratio of the three food types. Healthy eating leads to a balance of **roughly 50% carbohydrates, 25% protein, and 25% lipid** (fats and oils).

It is not necessary to spend a lot of time worrying about achieving those numbers. Simply continue to follow the guidelines through the lessons in the rest of the book and the goal will be achieved. We will provide the helpful numbers when we get to those topics, so that those of you who love to be analytical will have the details. You will also have your food plate as your guide.

You may have heard about 12-15 years ago that the ratio was "40-30-30". That was the science at the time and many programs that are being offered today are still based on those percentages. We don't quarrel with the actual numbers. The important detail is that somewhere around half of your daily calories come from a form of carbohydrate, and the other 50-60% is a balance of protein and lipids. In the meantime, perhaps the most helpful guideline as we get started is to remember to eat less each time and remember to eat more often. Maybe this thought will help. It certainly will prepare us for weeks 5-8.

1. Cut out all calories from beverages. That alone will   bring our carb calories into a healthier range.

2. Enjoy moderate servings of protein throughout the day. The good news is that we learn how to do that next week.

3. Eat real food. Get to know Michael Pollan, author of *Food Rules*. He advises, "If your great-grandmother wouldn't recognize it as food, don't eat it."

4. Shop around the perimeter of the grocery store. Choose healthy, live foods and the percentages will take care of themselves. (Week 8)

READ YOUR LABELS AND KEEP SCORE

Begin to pay closer attention to the information on food labels. 1% milk for instance, is 100 calories per glass. 48% carbohydrate, 28% protein, and 24% fat (lipids). We'll help you learn to figure some of that stuff out, at least enough to keep you healthy and happy

---

GET HEALTHY JOURNAL

Date:

"I maintain a healthy balance of the three food types."

HABIT 4: PLAN TO SUCCEED

What are some things that I have learned that will help me do a better job of eating "in balance"?

What seems to be the most helpful to keep me pointed in the right direction without all of this becoming complicated and confusing?

YOUR SCORE IS YOUR "THE EATER'S DIGEST"

WEEK 4 - DAY 5

"I will maintain a balance of healthy fats."

HABIT 5: NOURISH WITH REAL FOOD

Ann Louise Gittleman was our primary mentor and coach during the past 14 years. She has been one of the leaders in the field of nutritional sciences. She was one of the first researchers to discover in the early 1980s that the low fat movement was not only ineffective in terms of helping people lose weight, it was actually a dangerous way to eat. Book titles today, including hers, tell the story. The title of the book is "Eat Fat, Lose Weight".

Eating fat does not make us fat. Dietary fat (a form of lipid) is vital to health. The key is learning to distinguish between the unhealthy (man-made) fats and oils and those that the body needs but cannot produce so they are known as essential fats or essential fatty acids. While the name may be confusing it doesn't change the fact that healthy fat is good food.

This is perhaps, the trickiest part of the whole discussion we've had since the beginning. Some of the terms can get confusing. We acknowledge that. You see, we've been talking for almost four weeks about burning and losing fat and now we're learning that we need to eat more fat. If nothing else, let's find ways to simplify the topic.

For starters, let's remember that our goal is to eat real food or to eat as close to the natural food chain as possible. So even though we're going to devote the entire Week 7 to this topic, let's see if we can clear up a few things now. Here's a good look at the reasons that we need lipids (fats and oils) in our diet. This discussion is from our course titled "The Doctor's Plan for Healthy Eating".

The benefits of eating primarily healthy fats:

1. Fats are easily stored in the body and play a vital role in protecting the body from toxins.

2. Healthy (unsaturated) fats lower the levels of low-density lipoprotein (LDL), known as the "bad" cholesterol, without also lowering the levels of (HDL) or "good" cholesterol

3. They serve as a source of fuel for energy, beyond the quick energy that comes primarily from carbohydrates

4. Unsaturated fats reduce the development of erratic heartbeats, a main cause of cardiac death

5. Fats are an important constituent of the structure of all of the body's cells

6. Healthy fats reduce the tendency for blood clots to form in arteries

IDENTIFYING FATS

The key is to learn that the lipids that we get from plants and animals are NOT harmful when eaten in moderation. The "killer" fats that have made us weak and unhealthy for the past 100 years have now been labeled TRANS-fats and are gradually being removed from our foods. For now, begin by working on your thoughts and attitudes about this topic. Read this lesson several times, and certainly feel free to skip ahead to Week 7 and learn as much as you can. There are only three food types. It makes no sense to eliminate any one of them.

◆————————————————————◆

GET HEALTHY JOURNAL

Date:

"I will maintain a balance of healthy fats."

HABIT 5: NOURISH WITH REAL FOOD

What am I likely to think and say when I talk about fat in my foods?

Based on this information, does this make sense or do I need to re-think my understanding of this food type?

Am I willing to adjust my thinking?

EATING FAT DOES NOT MAKE US FAT

WEEK 4 - DAY 6

"I will embrace the most important concept in fat-burning."

HABIT 6: MOVE TO ACTIVATE YOUR METABOLISM

As always, we begin with the basics. Today you'll learn the introduction to what the world is just re-discovering as the simplest, yet most effective refinement in exercise of our time. You will learn what is known as **short-duration interval (SDI)** training. Let's get moving.

Begin by choosing your favorite form of movement. For about 70% of us, walking is a good place to start, but you may apply SDI to jogging, exercise machines, swimming, rebounding, or any form of activity. After a brief warm up of breathing, stretching, and Master Motions, you will begin the first phase of this training by doing one minute of exertion followed by one minute of recovery.

Our example is an 11-minute walking activity:

- Warm up, followed by one minute of brisk walking.

- At the end of a minute, slow to an easy walk and breathe deeply for a minute.

- Now, pick up the pace for one minute followed by another minute of recovery.

- The third set you will push yourself at a faster pace, perhaps causing you to tire a bit at the end of the minute.

- Another minute of recovery, followed by an intense minute where you push yourself at a very fast pace.

- Minute number eight is another segment of recovery followed by a minute of brisk walking

- Then another recover, and finally some time to "cool down.

As you can imagine, a stationary bicycle or a treadmill is an excellent application of this principle.

We'll learn more about this but for now learn to apply the SDI training once or twice each day, and be ready for more of those unwanted pounds to melt away. Even a short set of SDI training has shown to ignite fat-burning almost immediately. We now know that thermogenesis (fat-burning) continues for 3-5 hours after the activity is finished.

YOUR SDI TRAINING

Pick a time and a place where you can do SDI for about 10-15 minutes. Depending on the weather, you should not have to change clothing. It is one of the best ways to activate during the day, even during a short break at work. As is often the case, the main change is really just a change in your thinking. It is not necessary (or even desirable) to exert for a long period. High-intensity, short duration is the key.

After a few days of learning this activity, go for variety. Try another form of movement and apply the same principles. A detailed guide is available www.gethealthyandloseweight.com.

◆━━━━━━━━━━━━━━━━━━━━━━━━━◆

GET HEALTHY JOURNAL

Date:

"I will embrace the most important concept in fat-burning."

HABIT 6: MOVE TO ACTIVATE YOUR METABOLISM

What activity is the most simple for me to use in SDI training?

What other activity could I add for variation.

GET THERMOGENESIS WORKING FOR YOU

WEEK 4 - DAY 7

Today is a break day

HABIT 7: REFRESH TO STRENGTHEN YOUR COMMITMENT

You have been learning these habits one day at a time. If you are just looking to pick some "low-hanging fruit" that's OK. There will come a time when you will actually apply each lesson consecutively. 15 years of a lot of trial and tears have shown that's the way it works best. You have now devoted four full weeks to this effort, you certainly do deserve a break today, and perhaps a break for several days. Then, take some time to review each of the Habits and what you have learned.

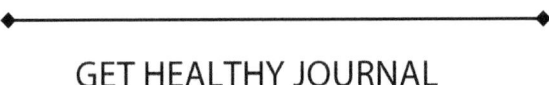

GET HEALTHY JOURNAL

Date:

Which habits will be the most important for me?

How has this journey changed my life up to this point?

AS I FORM NEW HABITS THEY WILL FORM THE NEW ME

.

PART II

WEEK 5- WEEK 8

HABITS 8-10 ARE ALL ABOUT FOOD

The second half of this guidebook is all about food. We've now begun the process of learning and developing healthier eating habits. Your compliance to these habits will grow over time as you practice and apply what you've learned. Learning the habits first provides a good, solid foundation upon which to learn the facts about the three types of food.

Our topic now becomes nutrition and the best definition of nutrition that we know is "the science of food and its relationship to health". Food is made up of a wide variety of nutrients, each of which has a very specific metabolic effect on the human body. Some of these nutrients are defined as **essential** while others are considered to be **non-essential**.

Essential nutrients are nutrients that cannot be synthesized (produced) by the human body and therefore must be derived from the food that we eat and digest. Essential nutrients include vitamins, minerals, amino acids, fatty acids and some carbohydrates as a source of energy. They **must** come from the food that we eat. Non-essential nutrients are nutrients which the body has the ability to create from other compounds in the body, as well as from food sources.

Nutrients are also generally divided into 2 categories, macronutrients, and micronutrients. Macronutrients constitute the majority of an individual's diet, thereby supplying energy, and the essential nutrients that are needed for growth, maintenance, and activity. The most common way of identifying foods as **"macro"** is that they are measured and thought of in ounces or grams. Macronutrients include carbohydrates, proteins, fats, macro minerals, and water. Carbohydrates, proteins, and fats are interchangeable as sources of energy in the body, with fats yielding 9 calories per gram, and protein and carbohydrates each yielding 4 calories per gram.

Micronutrients are vitamins and more than 60 minerals that are commonly referred to as "trace" minerals. Vitamins and trace minerals are labeled as micronutrients because the body only requires them in very small amounts. Macronutrients, as we've just learned are measured in ounces and/or grams, while micronutrients are listed as milligrams or even micrograms.

Vitamins are organic (living) substances that we ingest with our foods, and that "act as catalysts, substances that help to trigger other reactions in the body". Trace minerals are inorganic (meaning they are not living in the food but must be contained in the soil in which the food grows). These are important substances that once ingested play a role in a "variety of metabolic processes, and contribute to the synthesis of such elements as glycogen, protein, and fats".

Ron & Julie Meiss

WEEK 5 - DAY 1

"I am learning the value of lean, clean protein."

HABIT 8: FUEL WITH PROTEIN FOR STRENGTH

This healthy eating course was first drafted and taught in late 1996. As you can imagine, during that 15-year period the look and feel of the learning materials has changed dramatically. We have offered three-day jump starts and 7-day quick starts. Our most popular introductory offering has most often been taught as a 15-day turnaround. Depending on your first awareness of these materials, there's a very good chance that you've experienced one of those starter courses.

What has not changed is the overall content. We've always found that the key was to begin with a look at eating habits, and then turn our attention to understanding food and beverage and the role that they play in determining our overall health. No surprise then, that as we get to week 5, we begin to focus on food. Each lesson this week discusses protein. The word protein means "of first quality", and of the three food types, protein is the one that is needed on a daily basis. So, first we'll answer the basic question.... what is protein?

If you look at the parts of your body that you can see...your hair, your skin, your nails and your muscles...all are mostly protein. If you could look inside, the same would be true. The hemoglobin in your blood, the enzymes that keep us alive and active, and all of the hormones that we are learning about are made up of protein. There's no need to get overly technical here, but the building blocks of protein are some 20 amino acids. Because the body is constantly using protein, and because **we don't store amino acids** like we do essential fatty acids, there is an on-going need to replenish the body's supply of protein. How much protein do we need in a day?

There are a number of different guidelines to find the answer to the amount question and most of them involve grams and kilograms. A very simple method of figuring your protein need each day is to figure your approximate ideal weight and divide by two. For example, if your healthy weight is 140 pounds, divide by two for a suggested total of 70 grams. That means that an ideal day would be about 20-25 grams of protein at each of your three main meals and perhaps a few more grams as part of your snack or mini-meals. Your healthy breakfast choices are a nice fit in this formula and a 3-4 ounce serving of your favorite lean meat would also equal 20-25 grams. A typical serving of dairy provides about 8 grams and a large egg is about 6 grams. We'll give you some exact numbers on Day 3 this week, and even though this may seem a bit analytical right now, you will quickly learn why getting the right amount of protein each day is important..

YOUR NEED FOR PROTEIN

Begin with your ideal weight. Divide that number by two. You now have the number of grams of protein that your body can easily burn each day.

Make sure that you get protein at each of your meals, especially breakfast. The protein-fiber combinations or a healthy protein shake will provide a filling 15-20 grams. For a protein shake we suggest whey protein concentrate as the first ingredient of the powder that you use. For suggestions, visit our website.

BENEFITS

- If you are using protein shakes, whey protein (concentrate, rather than isolate) is an easily digestible source of all of the amino acids. There are definite benefits from choosing the whole food (concentrate) form of whey rather than a type that has been separated into selected pieces (isolate).

- Protein activates the hormone "glucagon", known as the fat-burning hormone.

EATING PROTEIN CREATES GLUCAGON,

THE FAT-BURNING HORMONE

WEEK 5 - DAY 2

"I eat protein throughout the day to avoid feeling hungry."

HABIT 8: FUEL WITH PROTEIN FOR STRENGTH

The best news of all this week is that protein throughout the day helps the body shed pounds quickly. The reasons include:

1. High-quality protein slows the movement of food from the stomach to the intestine. Slower stomach emptying means that you feel full for longer and are less likely to experience cravings.

2. Protein's rather gentle, steady effect on blood sugar helps avoid the rapid rise and fall that occurs after eating rapidly-digesting carbohydrates like white bread or a baked potato. The steady addition of protein throughout the day keeps the body in balance. There's even more good news:

The key for maintaining healthy weight loss is to **build muscle** with protein and activity, rather than **lose muscle** by denying yourself or eating poorly. Most diets may help you lose fat for a while, but you will also lose weight from your muscles, bones, heart, liver, intestines and kidneys which you do not want to lose.

Losing weight by not eating or **skipping meals causes loss of lean tissue and reduces the ability to burn calories**. This makes it more and more difficult to lose weight and/or to keep it off. By eating the right way during weight loss (which includes getting protein throughout the day), the body burns stored fat and protects the muscles allowing you to keep losing weight...and preventing the fat from coming back.

Later on we will teach you how to identify and add lean protein to your daily intake to keep you feeling satisfied and to keep building lean muscle. But before we finish today, let's make sure that we have an understanding. **We are not teaching a high-protein eating plan.** This formula presents a balanced eating plan with 20-25% of your daily calories coming in the form of protein. As we learn more about food, you'll appreciate this balance.

PROTEIN BREAKFAST AND SNACKS

Begin each day with 15-20 grams of protein for breakfast. That will be easy with a whey protein shake breakfast and can also be achieved with protein-fortified cereals. Our favorite is KASHI Go Lean. Other breakfast protein choices are to combine eggs, dairy, and lean meat with a fiber rich carbohydrate.

A great way to get an ounce or two of protein during the day or even as an evening snack is to add a small scoop of whey protein concentrate to a milk beverage.

BENEFITS

- You'll find it much easier to avoid feeling hungry throughout the day.

- Balance the body's blood sugar during the day (and the night) by replenishing protein.

- Some amino acids are "essential" meaning that they must be eaten regularly because they are not produced by the body. Keep the "building blocks" in ready supply.

THIS IS A BALANCED PROTEIN EATING PLAN

WEEK 5 - DAY 3

"I am learning a variety of ways to get plenty of healthy protein."

HABIT 8: FUEL WITH PROTEIN FOR STRENGTH

Many people are familiar with calculating the approximate number of calories they need per day. For instance, if you are an average-size woman weighing between 125-150, you might want to consume around 1500 calories. There are many different tools available on the internet if you would like to get more deeply into the topic, and if you choose to go for an easier calculation, take your weight times 10 for a woman and times 11 for a man to determine your "basal metabolic rate". That simply means the approximate amount of calories needed to maintain your current weight. If more detail would be helpful for you, visit our website http://gethealthyandloseweight.com/ and contact us at the address listed there.

If you take in around 1,500 calories a day and are aiming for 20-25% protein, you would need approximately 80 grams of protein a day. If you were trying to get 15% of your calories from protein, the daily total would be 65 grams of protein. Today we'll provide just a few daily examples of ways to figure your protein:

- 4 ounces ground sirloin, broiled = 30 grams protein

- 4 ounces pork tenderloin, roasted = 25 grams protein

- 4 ounces salmon, broiled = 29 grams protein

- 1 cup nonfat milk = 8 grams protein

- 1 cup light vanilla soy milk = 6 grams protein

- 1 ounce reduced fat cheese = 7 grams protein

- 1 ounce soy cheese (mozzarella) = 6 grams protein

- 1/2 cup of beans = about 7 grams protein

- 1/2 cup fresh green soybeans = 16 grams protein

- 3 ounces extra firm tofu = 8 grams protein

- 2 egg whites (1/4 cup egg substitute) = 7 grams protein

- 6 ounces yogurt = 5 grams protein

- 1 cup of broccoli = 4 grams protein

- 3/4 cup whole grain cereal = approx. 6 grams protein

- 12 ounce whey concentrate blended meal = 20 grams protein

- 3 ounces roasted chicken breast without skin = 26 grams protein

ANALYZE YOUR PROTEIN INTAKE

Take some time before going to bed tonight and take a look at your approximate protein intake. Remember that a good number to shoot for is about one-half of your ideal body weight in grams of protein.

Be sure that you include what we know as the plant proteins. Take a look at the list above and determine which ones are plant proteins. We'll learn more about those healthy foods tomorrow.

BENEFITS

- The numbers that we are learning in these lessons do not change. Once you've learned these "life-giving" principles they will allow you to eat healthy for the rest of your life.

- A tasty protein bar makes an excellent snack. Since we are always looking for mini-meal or snack ideas to fill in the mid-morning and mid-afternoon gaps, look for at least 10 grams of protein with a minimum amount of sugars and fats. Find suggestions at our website.

LEARN TO ENJOY PROTEIN WITH EACH MEAL

WEEK 5 - DAY 4

"I always look for ways to add plants, beans, and nuts to my plan."

HABIT 8: FUEL WITH PROTEIN FOR STRENGTH

Not long ago the nutritional thinking was that only animal sources of protein were valuable. Today vegetable sources of protein are not only recognized as lean and clean, they are also recommended as essential to good health. As prevention against cancer, heart disease, obesity, and diabetes, vegetable protein sources have become a cornerstone for healthy eating.

Animal protein sources including meat, dairy, and eggs provide all of the essential amino acids, but they are also high in saturated fats. We now know that when the animals that provided that protein were fed in a healthy way (grass-fed or range-fed) the fat contained healthier lipids and was beneficial for health. We'll cover this is much greater detail in two weeks. Many plant foods also contain protein, but most except fermented soy lack one or more essential amino acids which are the building blocks of protein.

By eating a variety of vegetable source proteins, one can obtain the complete range of amino acids and recommended daily protein.

Vegetable proteins also supply essential fats, complex carbohydrates, and fiber. Convenient vegetable protein powders are also available.

Combine grains, nuts and seeds, which are lacking in the amino acid lysine, with legumes which have lysine. Combine legumes, which are lacking in the amino acid methionine, with grains and nuts to balance out that need. **Vegetable Protein Sources are:**

- Grains (lacking in lysine): brown rice, rye, wheat, cornmeal, barley, millet, oats, buckwheat

- Nuts and Seeds (lacking in lysine): walnuts, cashews, almonds, pecans, sunflower seeds, pumpkin seeds, sesame seeds, flax seeds, hemp seeds

- Legumes (lacking in methionine): beans, peas, lentils, garbanzos (chickpeas) and Soy products

BASIC GUIDELINES TO COMPLEMENTING PROTEINS

Combine legumes and grains. Examples include rice and beans (black or kidney beans, lentils, or black-eyed peas) Tortillas and beans, barley and bean soup, or a peanut butter sandwich with whole grain bread.

Combine legumes and nuts or seeds. Examples include Hummus chickpeas with sesame paste, bean soup with sesame seeds or other nuts, or combine beans, chickpeas, and various nuts in a salad.

BENEFITS

- Vegetable proteins are a great source of complex carbohydrates, essential minerals, a variety of the essential fatty acids and are the best food source of dietary fiber.

- Plant sources of complete proteins are: spirulina, quinoa, buckwheat, hempseed, and amaranth, & soy products such as soybeans, tofu, tempeh, and miso.

THEN GOD SAID, "I GIVE YOU EVERY SEED-BEARING PLANT ON THE FACE OF THE EARTH AND EVERY TREE THAT HAS FRUIT WITH SEED IN IT. THEY WILL BE YOURS FOR FOOD."

GENESIS 1:29

WEEK 5 - DAY 5

"A protein shake makes perfect sense with my busy life."

HABIT 8: FUEL WITH PROTEIN FOR STRENGTH

Most health experts agree that breakfast is clearly the most important meal of the day. You have enjoyed a healthy breakfast for the past few weeks, and you are experiencing the benefits of feeling satisfied all morning long. Most of your early morning meals and even some of your other daily meals have come in the form of a tasty "nourishment" that we call a blended meal.

We recently spoke with a group of healthy-weight coaches and asked their response to the consumption of whey-based meals. Here are the top five benefits mentioned:

1. **Energy** – protein plus other healthy added nutrients creates long-lasting energy.

2. **Convenience** – using a top-quality shaker, it's easy to fit a protein shake into a busy lifestyle.

3. **Nutrition** – biologically active whey protein concentrate enhances health, especially the immune system.

4. **Taste** – Whey shakes mixes can usually be found in great tasting flavors.

5. **Cost** – These tasty meals often cost less than $2 a meal making a wonderful value.

The idea mentioned most often was to have a shaker with you at all times or keep one at home and one at work. There are so many valuable nutrients available in powder form today including vitamin D and you can easily add any of them to a convenient blended meal.

It is clear that the biggest challenge for most of us is getting used to the fact that we can have a complete meal in the form of a tasty shake. We've mentioned this before....the biggest factor may be your decision to stop for a moment, relax, and enjoy. If you find yourself drinking too quickly, take time for some relaxing breathing between sips.

PROTEIN SHAKES

Look for additional items that can be added to a blended meal. Try some different forms of fiber, cinnamon, or other powdered nutrients at the healthy food store.

Always be sure to shake the blend thoroughly, and then let it settle for a few minutes. Allow time for the nutrients to dissolve and blend before consuming.

BENEFITS

- A wonderful, quick way to get your daily vitamins, minerals and other nutrients.

- Having a quick blended meal available supports healthy blood sugar levels all day long.

- Provides a lean, clean, easily-digestible source of protein.

A WHOLE FOOD "SMOOTHIE" WITH PROTEIN
MAKES A BALANCED MEAL

WEEK 5 - DAY 6

"I look for ways to find quality protein ."

HABIT 8: FUEL WITH PROTEIN FOR STRENGTH

We have now spent a week together learning about proteins, the type of food upon which our bodies are built. Interestingly, there has been comparatively little study done on protein and so we still have a lot to learn. Continue to find creative ways to use a high-quality whey concentrate as the base for some tasty blended meals and you'll have up to ½ of your daily requirements covered. There is also a lot more to learn about other healthy protein snacks such as bars and cookies which are also continuing to improve in both texture and taste.

Before we move on to learn more about the other two food types, let's talk just a bit more about some important factors involving animal proteins. You may not have spent much time yet thinking about today's topic, but the diet of the animals that are the source of our protein has a major impact on the nutritional quality, safety, and healthfulness of the food that we get from them. This is true of the eggs, the dairy products, and the meat that we consume as a part of our daily diet.

As you think about this, it will likely be self-evident, and yet it really doesn't seem to matter to the decision-makers of the giant food manufacturing companies who are looking for ways to produce and provide huge supplies of low-cost animal protein. We will choose to stay out of the politics of this important question, and simply say that the pursuit of cheap sources of these important foods has drastically changed the diet of these food animals and is clearly damaging to their health and to ours.

In every case, these animals are much healthier when they are able to have access to green plants and grasses for their food, and so are the meat, dairy and eggs that they produce. It is well worth some of your time to become more knowledgeable on these issues. There are many books, articles and other resources that address this important topic. We can summarize our thinking by saying that it is always good to look for foods from animals that are "pastured," "free range," or "hormone free."

STUDY THE SOURCE

Begin by looking at the eggs available where you shop for food. Ask about organic, range-fed, or even eggs as a source of "healthy fats". More about omega-3 fatty acids in a few days.

It might be a good idea to familiarize yourself with sources of dairy, meat and eggs that are produced "locally". The same providers will provide you with access to other valuable food sources. Here's an example of one of our favorites as of Summer 2011:

"LocalHarvest is an organic and local food website. We maintain a definitive and reliable "living" public nationwide directory of small farms, farmers markets, and other local food sources. Our search engine helps people find products from family farms, local sources of sustainably grown food, and encourages them to establish direct contact with small farms in their local area." – www.localharvest.org

BENEFITS

- Animals that eat healthy are a much higher quality source of food for human consumption.

- Buying locally and learning more about your food sources, will result in a fresher food supply than those mass-produced foods at the super market.

- Saturated fats from grass-fed animals contain higher levels of CLA, a healthy fat that is vital to the digestion of all forms of fat in the body.

EAT PROTEIN FROM ANIMALS THAT ATE HEALTHY FOOD

WEEK 5 - DAY 7

Today is a break day

HABIT 7: REFRESH TO STRENGTHEN YOUR COMMITMENT

Our experience has taught us that this is a good time to have a brief heart-to-heart talk. We have carefully crafted this guidebook so that it can be "digested" one day at a time for a period of eight weeks. We find that fewer than one in five participants actually use the book that way. Most get so engrossed in the process that they read a little sometime and then a lot of pages over a weekend, for example. **That is perfectly OK.**

You're an adult and you paid for this information. The thing that is important to us is that you find these ideas to be useful, that you are doing a better job of healthy eating, and you are moving in the direction of a healthier lifestyle. Most importantly, today is a break day. Go out and enjoy your time with those you love

THE WISE MAN SHOULD CONSIDER THAT HEALTH IS THE GREATEST OF HUMAN BLESSINGS. LET FOOD BE YOUR MEDICINE "
- HIPPOCRATES

WEEK 6 - DAY 1

"I eat at least 50% of my calories from carbs."

HABIT 9: FUEL WITH CARBOHYDRATES FOR ENERGY

Our food lessons continue here in week six with a closer look at what is by far the largest of the three food types, the foods that we will come to know as carbohydrates. To begin this learning, please go back and review Week 3 – Day 5 where you were first introduced to grains. Today we'll focus once again on grains.

Often referred to as the "staff of life" for their historical importance to human survival, grains are an essential part of a healthy diet. Also called cereals, grains are the seeds of grasses, which are cultivated for food. The important thing to remember is that grains should be eaten in their "whole" form rather than processed. These are the keys to insuring that you are eating grain in its intended form.

Refined Foods – often used to describe any type of processed food. Processing grains means the grains have been stripped of their nutrient value by a chemical process. Bleach is then used to make the flour white.

Wheat bread is usually not whole wheat - Be aware when you are looking at "wheat bread". A closer look will reveal that it has the same basic ingredients as the white bread on the shelf next to it. It simply has caramel coloring added to make it brown in color.

Don't be fooled by the term, "enriched flour", because typically, only four vitamins and minerals are added back, compared to the 15 that are lost, along with most of the fiber and other beneficial substances like antioxidants. Whole-grain versions of rice, bread, cereal, flour and pasta can be found at any grocery store.

Always go "light on white"- Refined grains, such as white rice or white flour, have both the bran and germ removed from the grain. Although vitamins and minerals are added back into refined grains after the milling process, they still don't have as many nutrients as whole grains do, and they don't provide as much fiber naturally.

Enriched Wheat Flour and Fortified Wheat Flour are not healthy – This means that it is highly-processed white flour that it is missing the two most nutritious and fiber-rich parts of the seed: the outside bran layer and the germ (embryo). Eating this "white" empty by-product can leave the body malnourished, constipated, enervated (weakened) and vulnerable to chronic illness.

Know Your Grams - A slice of commercially prepared white bread has 66 calories, 1.9 grams protein and 0.6 grams fiber. A slice of whole-wheat bread has 69 calories and provides 3.6 grams protein and 1.9 grams fiber. **Choose grains with at least 3 grams of dietary fiber per serving whenever possible.**

HOW MUCH GRAIN TO EAT

Your goal is to eat at least two healthy servings of grains per day. Eat one serving of whole-grain cereal or toast with your protein for breakfast. If you haven't already thought of this, it's a good time to remember that the easiest way to get a good healthy grain is with a bowl of your favorite oatmeal. Here are two suggestions:

Oatmeal, flaxseed, blueberries & almonds. Steel-cut oatmeal is probably the healthier choice, but if you are in a hurry, the instant kind will do fine (especially the kinds that have added fiber and protein). Heat the water – stir in the oatmeal, add ground flaxseed, frozen blueberries, sliced almonds. You can add a little cinnamon and honey (not a lot) if you're using the non-instant oatmeal. That's four power foods, full of fiber and nutrients and protein and good fats, with only a couple of minutes of prep time.

Kashi Golean crunch (also available as a hot cereal). Actually, any whole-grain, high-fiber cereal with added protein is a good choice, this just happens to be one of our favorites. It has a high amount of protein and fiber, low sugar. Add low-fat milk or soy milk (which has 1/3 the saturated fat of 1% milk), and perhaps some berries if you like.

BENEFITS

- Grain is an excellent source of fiber. Choose cereal and bread that is high in fiber.

- When eaten whole, grain is also an important contribution to daily protein intake.

THE WHITER THE BREAD THE QUICKER YOU'RE DEAD

WEEK 6 - DAY 2

"I am learning the benefits of eating 'foods of many colors'."

HABIT 9: FUEL WITH CARBOHYDRATES FOR ENERGY

One of our favorite mentors (Dr. Ann Louise Gittelman) has always advised that we should "eat all the colors of the rainbow". Fruits are very colorful, and you'll also realize just how many vegetables are full of color. Most of the life-giving nutrients are contained in the part of the food which also gives it its color. Fruits and vegetables are two of the major groups of foods that are also carbohydrates. We'll also learn this week that it is important to retain the color by eating the food raw or as close to fresh as possible. That may mean frozen or lightly steamed and it will never mean canned or "over-cooked".

These ideas might encourage you to eat more of the fruits and vegetables available to you:

- They have a high content of water just like the human body.

- Fruits and vegetables contain none of the harmful type of cholesterol.

- Most of these colorful foods are filled with fiber.

- The color in the healthy carbohydrates contains many of the healthy micronutrients .

These healthy foods can actually make you feel better and provide constant energy throughout the day.

Here's an important key to healthy eating. Any one of the fruits and vegetables that we will be discussing contains dozens, in fact likely hundreds of different phytonutrients that have an important effect on the body. As you will quickly see, the benefits go far beyond the obvious which is increased energy. You also need to know that no single fruit or vegetable contains all of the substances that the body needs. That's why it's a good idea to get a few servings a week from each of the major groups.

GET ENOUGH FRUITS AND VEGETABLES

Add lots of extra and colorful fresh vegetables to a dinner salad. Add a variety of frozen fruits to a whey protein shake to greatly enhance the taste.

Many health food stores sell packets of high-quality freeze-dried fruit and vegetable powders. Check out consuming one each day to fill the nutritional gaps.

BENEFITS

- Help you feel full with fewer calories

- Lower blood pressure

- Help avoid constipation and diverticulitis

- Delay or prevent memory loss and a decline in thinking skills

- Decrease the chances of having a heart attack or stroke

EAT ALL THE COLORS OF THE RAINBOW

WEEK 6 - DAY 3

"I always choose fresh or frozen before canned."

HABIT 9: FUEL WITH CARBOHYDRATES FOR ENERGY

Eat your fruits and vegetables. **Vegetable -** Any vegetable or 100% vegetable juice is a member of the "colorful carbohydrate" group. Vegetables may be raw or cooked; fresh, frozen, canned, or dried/dehydrated; and they may be whole, cut-up, or mashed. Some vegetables are more than 70% water and are very important to proper hydration.

Fruits - Any fruit or 100% fruit juice counts as part of the fruit group. Fruits may be fresh, canned, frozen, or dried, and may be whole, cut-up, or pureed. When we are talking about healthy eating, a **fruit** is the part of the plant that contains its seeds

Vegetables: Eat all you will. Notice we did not say all you can.

- **Raw is best.** The body loves raw or live foods. Fresh vegetables are available all year long and are easy to clean and enjoy. You can even find little "snack packs" in the produce section and enjoy them at any time.

- **Frozen is a good choice.** The frozen food section of your favorite store has a great selection of vegetables. These foods were picked and frozen quickly and contain all of the nutrients that are found in fresh.

- **Steam Lightly** - When preparing vegetables for a meal, you will find it easy to use the frozen kind and simply steam them lightly to maintain the enzymes.

- **Canned is seldom a good choice.** Most foods lose their freshness when canned and some of the cans may even introduce unhealthy chemicals into the contents.

- **Avoid the microwave when preparing fresh foods**. More on that later.

Fruits: Eat fruit at least twice a day – preferably by itself. Fruit digests very quickly and can be trapped in the stomach as proteins and other foods linger longer. It's best to have a nice serving of fruit by itself.

- **Enjoy fruit fresh** and especially when in-season.

- **Avoid Canned Fruit** - It is usually packed with added sugar.

- **Consume fruit juice in small amounts**. A fruit juice glass is only four ounces. Processed juices have the fiber stripped and are a potent source of fructose (sugar).

- **Freshly squeezed juices are much healthier.** Especially if you juice them yourself. Processed fruit juice (bottle, can or box) often contains only about 10% fruit juice. The package must contain the % information. Choose 100% fruit juice.

EAT YOUR FRUIT

Enjoy fruit as a snack or mini-meal or in small amounts with a meal. Fruit is best when eaten alone. Grapes, melon, berries and other colorful "carbs" make a great snack and even a dessert.

As a child, you learned about "an apple a day". Beginning today, add an apple, peach, pear or plum as a regular routine for one of your snacks. An added benefit is a healthy serving of that dietary fiber that most of us can always use more of.

BENEFITS

- Fruits and vegetable (eaten live) are an excellent source of hydration, adding up to a full glass of beverage to your daily total.

- Add variety to your food choices and awaken your taste buds.

A FRUIT JUICE GLASS HOLDS ONLY 4 OUNCES FOR A REASON

WEEK 6 - DAY 4

"I try to consume at least 30-35 grams of fiber each day."

HABIT 9: FUEL WITH CARBOHYDRATES FOR ENERGY

Dietary fiber — found mainly in fruits, vegetables, whole grains and legumes (all of which are your healthy carbohydrates) — is probably best known for its ability to prevent or relieve constipation. But fiber can provide other health benefits as well, such as lowering your risk of diabetes and heart disease. Selecting tasty foods that provide fiber isn't difficult.

Dietary fiber, also known as roughage or bulk, includes all parts of plant foods that your body can't digest or absorb. Unlike other food components such as fats, proteins or carbohydrates — which your body breaks down and absorbs — fiber isn't digested by your body. Therefore, it passes relatively intact through your stomach, small intestine, colon and out of your body.

It might seem like fiber doesn't do much, but it has several important roles in maintaining health. Fiber is commonly classified into two categories: those that don't dissolve in water (insoluble fiber) and those that do (soluble fiber).

Insoluble fiber. This type of fiber promotes the movement of material through your digestive system and increases stool bulk, so it can be of benefit to those who struggle with constipation or irregular stools. Whole-wheat flour, wheat bran, nuts and many vegetables are good sources of insoluble fiber.

Soluble fiber. This type of fiber dissolves in water to form a gel-like material. It can help lower blood cholesterol and glucose levels. Soluble fiber is found in oats, peas, beans, apples, citrus fruits, carrots, barley and psyllium.

The amount of each type of fiber varies in different plant foods. To receive the greatest health benefit, eat a wide variety of high-fiber foods.

GET YOUR FIBER

Make sure that you find a way to get about 10 grams of fiber with breakfast. Add fiber to your smoothies or to your cereal.

Many of the newer breakfast bars contain fiber. Why not buy a box of FIBER ONE and try one.

BENEFITS

- **Normalizes bowel movements.** Dietary fiber increases the weight and size of your stool and softens it.

- **Lowers blood cholesterol levels.**

- **Helps control blood sugar levels and aids in weight loss.**

FIBER IS NOT DIGESTED - ITS PURPOSE IS TRANSPORTATION

WEEK 6 - DAY 5

"I look for opportunities to eat raw foods."

HABIT 9: FUEL WITH CARBOHYDRATES FOR ENERGY

Raw food means we are talking about fruit, nuts, berries and vegetables, and other "live" foods which taste good to the majority of people in their basic simple form, direct from tree, bush, or vine. Another way of describing this type of eating is to: "eat as close to the natural food chain as possible".

How Much Raw Food Should I eat? We realize it isn't easy or practical to simply abandon thousands of years of tradition and revert back to anything close to 100% raw food. Begin by thinking of 25-30% of your daily intake coming from live food. You will gradually learn to add more.

Don't eat raw meat.— Enjoy the freshest, leanest cuts of your favorites, cooked as you like. Grass or range fed is the best.

Are lightly cooked vegetables OK? Yes, learn to steam your vegetables, either fresh or frozen.

Raw foods offer better quality nutrition. You can eat less to satisfy your daily food needs. The heat of cooking depletes vitamins, damages proteins and fats, and destroys enzymes which benefit digestion.

Raw foods naturally have more flavor than cooked foods so there is no need to add salt, sugar, spices, or other condiments that can irritate your digestion system or over-stimulate other organs.

Raw foods take very little preparation so you spend less time in preparation. Every member of the family can pitch in and help prepare tasty, live foods.

Cleaning up after a raw meal is a snap. There are no baked-on oils or crusty messes. Any parts that are cut away are discarded and can go directly to the compost pile.

Eating raw saves money By choosing carefully you can save on food, cooking utensils, appliances, and possibly, even the expense of some doctor bills, drugs, and health insurance.

Get "Real" - Return to foods that are "natural"…food that comes from nature. Remember that there is no spring that flows with carbonated water; there are no Twinkie trees, and no Doritos plants. **The easiest raw foods to eat are** fruits, vegetables, nuts, berries, and sprouts.

EATING RAW

This may be a good time to go through your pantry and give away most of your canned goods. There may be a few exceptions, but most canned food is "dead". Nuts are an excellent source of raw foods. Pay close attention next week as we learn more about the different healthy lipids that are abundant in nuts and seeds.

Purchase a steamer basket and learn to lightly steam your vegetables for your evening meal. This will provide some variety as you learn to consume more of your food in its natural state. Steaming "lightly" allows the food to retain all of the enzymes and the other nutrients that are present when the plant is live. Look at recipes and learn to add spices and some real butter to add to the great taste.

BENEFITS

- **Better digestion** - Live foods contain the enzymes needed for digestion.

- **More energy** - Even from smaller meals

- **Improved skin appearance** – A result of the nutrients and the hydration

EAT AS CLOSE TO THE NATURAL FOOD CHAIN AS POSSIBLE

Week 6 - Day 6

"I will avoid added sweeteners in my food and drink ."

HABIT 9: FUEL WITH HEALTHY CARBOHYDRATES FOR ENERGY

As this latest edition of the guide book was being readied to go to print, the headlines in the major weekend media read, "Sugar's Shocking effects on Health". We started this week's lessons by discussing all of the issues regarding "white" flour. Today we'll end the week with a serious look at the other "white" culprit that is refined sugar. We'll begin with a very strong solution that you will want to develop into a daily habit.

Avoid added sweeteners. Get to know and avoid these harmful substances! **Recognize sugar in all of its forms.** Added sugar refers any sugar or sugar substitute that you or the manufacturer adds to the real food. We'll give you some help in a moment.

It is true that all food breaks down into sugar as the form of energy and life to our cells, but, excessive sugar and bad carb intake causes numerous health problems. You should become familiar with the following:

- **Learn to read labels**. anything that ends in **"ose"** is a form of sugar: fructose, maltose, sucrose, etc. There are more than 100 names for caloric sweeteners ranging from corn syrup to malted barley. They are all forms of added sugar. Learn to read labels and begin to recognize hidden sugars.

- **High fructose corn syrup** is a major problem and clearly the most popular sweetener on the market today. We'll go on record as saying that the research proves that it is the most "troubling" of all of the artificial sweeteners we have ever studied. And yes, it is artificial. The manufacturing process is very complex and creates a product that is certainly not healthy.

- **Watch high glycemic foods.** The glycemic index is a measurement for a particular food's effect on blood glucose (blood sugar). These are sugars and may be "bad" carbs.

Learn to calculate teaspoons of sugar per serving - Remember to notice the number of *servings* in the container. A 20-ounce bottle contains 2.5 servings and often a great deal of some form of sweetener. Here's the math:

6. 20-ounce bottle of tea with lemon

7. 2.5 servings per bottle (the label is based on 8 ounces)

8. Label reports 26 grams of sugar (per serving)

9. Total sugar in one bottle is 26x2.5=65 grams of sugar (about 16 teaspoons). **Can you imagine consuming 16 teaspoons of sugar at one sitting? You may be doing that many times per day!**

WATCH YOUR LABELS

As you consider beverage purchases, look at the label. Immediately replace any drink that contains High Fructose Corn Syrup. As we requested, go back and review the lesson from Week 3 – Day 2 Learn to look for healthier alternatives among the various types of sweeteners.

BENEFITS

1. **Avoiding bad food is making a huge improvement in your future health.** Eliminating or reducing certain highly-sweetened foods from your diet will have the biggest impact on your health. Taking bad stuff out of your diet might be more important than eating the good things.

2. **Many harmful substances are disguised.** You must stay on your toes to avoid their damage to you.

3. **Get to know your weakness.** We all have one or more. Growing into a healthy lifestyle starts with knowing your vulnerabilities.

WE REPEAT....DO NOT DRINK YOUR CALORIES

WEEK 6 - DAY 7

"Today is a break day."

HABIT 7: REFRESH TO STRENGTHEN YOUR COMMITMENT

We've promised you a break today and we want to honor that commitment. The week ahead will introduce us to the one remaining food type and then we have some "fun" sessions together in Week 8. As you relax and enjoy this day, spend a little time reflecting on some things that you've learned, especially about this food called "carbs". It's really silly that some people would consider going on a "low-carb" diet. Almost every real food that we pick up is a carbohydrate. The key is to know which ones we want to "pick up'

Go out and be blest.

"DON'T DIG YOUR GRAVE WITH YOUR OWN KNIFE AND FORK." -
ENGLISH PROVERB

Ron & Julie Meiss

WEEK 7 - DAY 1

"I eat 25% of my calories from Fats and Oils."

HABIT 10: FUEL WITH LIPIDS FOR NORMAL BODY FUNCTIONS

As we begin another week of lessons, we move to the third and final food type known as lipids usually referred to simply as fats (and oils). After more than 14 years of teaching these food lessons, we have clearly learned that this is the greatest subject of food confusion. Let's begin by getting some facts straight.

Some of the best people we have worked with have long said that as a result of all the mis-information of the past 30 years, we have become fat phobic. Talk to someone about weight loss and the first thing they may mention is eliminating fat from their diet. We have been taught that fat is bad, that fat is the enemy. Since sometime back in the mid-1970s, we have read about ways to slash the fat, cut the fat, lose the fat or, at least, lower the fat. Ask someone to look at a food label and the first thing they comment on is the percent or the grams of fat. Here is a very important fact.....**eating fat does not make you fat!**

Simply put, our bodies could not function without adequate fat. We'll continue to learn that at least 25% of our daily caloric intake should come from fat. The American Heart Association recommends up to 30%. Here are some of the main reasons:

Healthy fats nourish the skin, nerves, and mucous membranes; they strengthen the immune, cardiovascular, reproductive and central nervous systems; fats are required for the production of hormones; they facilitate oxygen transportation and calcium and other mineral absorption; fatty acids assist in the absorption of the fat soluble vitamins A, D E, and K and are critical for heart health. It all begins with the development of the infant brain which is comprised of more than 50% fat. The brain chemicals, we know them as *neurotransmitters,* are all regulated by hormones that are created from fat. As you continue to study nutrition, you will see that there really is no other nutrient available to us that can heal (heal is the root word of health) the entire body from birth to old age like the assortment of fatty acids available in our foods.

However, **all fats are not created equal.** The problem that we alluded to earlier is that we've been exposed to misguided and distorted information that has grouped all fats into in the same "bad" category. Remember, **fat is not the enemy**. Let's move forward with an open mind and reveal the truth to counter **the big "fat" lie**.

INTRODUCTION TO FATS

Realize that what you are about to learn will require some "unlearning". Commit to getting the real skinny about fat and finding ways to get the good stuff into your daily diet.

Mixed nuts are an excellent snack, provide lots of good fats and oils, and contribute to feeling satisfied or full. Purchase some quality mixed nuts for a snack each day this week.

BENEFITS

- Regular consumption of EFA (essential fatty acid) has been shown to improve good cholesterol.

- Healthy fat is a major contributor to the development of the immune system.

- Daily consumption of good fats allows the body to release stored bad fat.

HEALTHY FAT IS A FRIEND – NOT AN ENEMY

WEEK 7 - DAY 2

"I have started finding ways to go from good fats to better fats."

HABIT 10: FUEL WITH LIPIDS FOR NORMAL BODY FUNCTIONS

We're going to talk about some kinds of fats. Don't worry about understanding all of the talk about "polyunsaturated", "mono-unsaturated" and "lipids". Just concentrate on the fact that these healthy fats are good for you and the real key is to consume them in the correct balance.

Today we are focusing on what scientists know as a polyunsaturated fat and we have come to know as a linoleic acid (another term you don't have to remember) called **Omega-6.** The key to playing the fatty acid game is to find a way to eat them in the right amounts. Tomorrow we'll get acquainted with "Omega-3" and learn that the combination of Omega-6 and Omega-3 is what produces the health benefits that we've talked about.

Most of us are not deficient in Omega-3 as likely as we are overloaded with Omega-6. Here's why ... Remember that we are not saying that these Omega-6 oils should not be consumed. What we ARE saying is that in our agri-industrial society, there is way too much emphasis placed on corn and soybean oils along with all of the other products created as a result of these two grains. What further complicated the issue, was the introduction of hydrogenated and partially-hydrogenated oils made from corn and soybeans. The process is simply injecting a hydrogen molecule into the oil for better preservation. The problem is that this created a form of trans-fatty acid that we now know, is very harmful to our health. The good news is that we now clearly realize the dangers of these hydrogenated oils and they are gradually being removed from our food supply. For example: when is the last time that you bought margarine or shortening? Hopefully, those "killers" are gone from your shopping list.

The best and quickest way to reduce the amount of these fats and oils from your diet, is to cut back on the packaged **"C" foods**. These processed food-like substances include **Chips, Cookies, Crackers** and **sweetened Cereals.** Even though the lable says 0 trans fats, there is still a small amount allowed. (We'll say more on Day 5 this week.) Go for the real food instead. These processed and packaged food items do not encourage good health.

The best sources of Omega-6 are seeds, nuts, grains, green leafy vegetables and certain raw vegetable oils. Learn to use olive oil, sesame oil, Chia seed oil, or hempseed oil instead of always relying on the common vegetable oils. We'll learn more about olives and olive oil tomorrow.

HEALTHY FAT STRATEGIES

Look for seeds such as pumpkin seeds, sunflower seeds, and pine nuts to add to your healthy snacks. Raw nuts and seeds are a wonderful source of Omega-6.

Cut back on the amount of oil you eat in salad dressings. Begin today to order your salad dressing on the side. A tasty salad flavoring is meant to dress the salad, not drench it. Try dipping your fork in the little cup to add the desired amount of flavor and then add the salad to the fork. Your last taste will be the dressing.

BENEFITS

- A balance of Omega-6 and Omega-3 is critical for all systems of the body to function normally.

- Healthy fats are important to adding flavor to the food.

- 25% of daily calories from fat eliminates hungry times and reduces cravings.

UTIMATELY WE MUST EAT FAT TO BURN FAT

WEEK 7 - DAY 3

"I will acquire the health benefits of Omega-3 fatty acids."

HABIT 10: FUEL WITH LIPIDS FOR NORMAL BODY FUNCTIONS

I (Ron) was working for a major health food store in Phoenix, Arizona. A customer approached the counter and demanded to know: "If you could buy only one item in this store to maintain excellent health, what would it be?" Without hesitation, I walked with her in the direction of the **essential fatty acids (EFA)**. The point to remember is that Omega-3 EFA is vital to normal healthy functioning, and that it takes some thought and effort to achieve a good balance.

Omega-3 fatty acid (Alpha-linoleic) is very important for brain function and plays a major role in the prevention of cardiovascular disease. This essential fat which must be eaten, (it is not made in the body) plays a critical role in keeping the heart beating at a steady clip and not lapsing into dangerous, sometimes fatal erratic rhythms.

The American Heart Association recommends a diet in which fatty fish, like salmon, herring, sardines and tuna are consumed at least twice a week. Fish oil supplements are a good alternative if you don't like to eat fish, or if you've been warned about contamination. They are rich in EPA. You can protect against mercury and other concerns by choosing a quality gel cap that is contaminant-free.

Another of the most important functions of Omega-3 is to make up cell membranes throughout the body, especially the eye and the brain cells. They provide the starting point from which some hormones are made including the ones that regulate blood clotting, contraction and relaxation of artery walls and inflammation. It is quite easy to see the connection with aiding in the prevention of heart disease and stroke.

Let's talk about another fatty acid. Omega-9, or mono-saturated oleic and stearic acid, is a non-essential fatty acid produced naturally by the body when there is sufficient Omega-6 and Omega-3 present. It can also be a healthy addition to the diet in the form of olive and olive oil, "mixed" nuts such as pecans, cashews, almonds, pistachios, and macadamia, and is especially rich in avocados. Yes, that tasty, green fruit. Omega-9 plays an important role in this healthy fat issue due to its proven role in preventing heart disease by lowering cholesterol levels and reducing hardening of the arteries. All Omega fatty acids play a key role in improving immune function.

HEALTHY FAT STRATEGIES

Look for ways to increase your intake of fatty fish, or add a high-quality fish oil supplement to your daily routine.

Notice that we've been talking about mixed nuts all week. Find a good mixture that contains sea salt. Often available at your local Costco or Sam's Club. Mixed nuts are great source of your Omegas.

BENEFITS

- EFAs are now known to play a key role in reducing occurrences of the "itis" diseases – rheumatoid arthritis, bursitis, colitis, dermatitis, gingivitis, and bronchitis.

- Physicians who practice "complementary" medicine, often recommend Omega-3 supplements for immune-related diseases.

ALL OMEGA FATTY ACIDS IMPROVE IMMUNE FUNCTION

WEEK 7 - DAY 4

"I will use excellent sources of healthy saturated fat."

HABIT 10: FUEL WITH LIPIDS FOR NORMAL BODY FUNCTIONS

We've said since the beginning that our biggest obstacle in learning to eat healthy is confusion. We asked at the beginning of these lessons on lipids that you would keep an open mind. Today we are going to ask you to consider this lesson on saturated fat, do some research on your own, making sure that you are tapped into the latest and most accurate reports. Then, make a decision for yourself regarding your personal intake of saturated fat. The good news is that all scientific literature recommends somewhere between 7% and 10% of your daily fat intake come in the form of saturated fats. So let's begin our discussion today with some ideas.

Nuts: We've recommended mixed nuts as a good source of many of the types of fat, including saturated fat. We trust that you are learning that one of the major benefits of consuming at least 25% of your daily intake of calories in the form of fat is a wonderful feeling of satiety, or what one of our researchers calls feeling "comfortably full". Nuts and seeds are an excellent source of saturated fats.

Coconut oil: This healthy, tropical oil has been put down for many years due to concerns about the amount of saturated fat. Today we realize that there are many health benefits derived from this lipid which is most accurately called medium-chain fatty acid. In addition to skin and hair care, **pure virgin coconut oil** provides a metabolic boost for weight loss.

Grass-fed meats: Remember the lesson on proteins. Now is the time to review how to improve the quality of the proteins in your diet. Ironically, by choosing better sources of protein, you will completely change the make-up of the fats found in the meat, dairy and eggs that you consume. This is obviously a much deeper topic than we can cover today, but we do encourage you to learn about the benefits of choosing food from animals that have been grass fed. The animal's digestive systems were meant to feed on grasses, not corn and soy. A whole new world of health awaits you.

MORE HEALTHY FAT STRATEGIES

Begin to add some coconut oil to your blended meals. Notice how it adds to the fresh taste and increases your sense of fullness for a longer period of time.

Consider purchasing a better quality of milk. At least make sure that it is free of added hormones and try the 1% variety. You're adding back some saturated fat and creating a near-perfect ratio of the three food types.

BENEFITS

- 60% of the makeup of the brain is saturated fat. All of the body's cellular membrane is made up entirely of fat.

- The suggestion that saturated fat is damaging to health is not supported by scientific literature.

HEALTHY FAT = HEALTHY SKIN, HEALTHY HAIR & HEALTHY NAILS

WEEK 7 - DAY 5

"I will work at eliminating all of the bad fats ."

HABIT 10: FUEL WITH LIPIDS FOR NORMAL BODY FUNCTIONS

Hopefully, we will soon see the day when this lesson may no longer be necessary. The word is quickly getting out that there is no place in our diet for trans-fats which are usually identified as hydrogenated or partially-hydrogenated oils. This false food, created in Germany in 1901 to keep oils from going bad, is detrimental to human health and must be avoided. The National Academy of Sciences says that there is no safe quantity that can be consumed. The good news is that food manufacturers and even most restaurants are being much more careful about using trans fats in order to serve today's health-conscious public.

There are currently at least five ways that you can still get trapped. Watch for these "traps" and you can eliminate these "killer" fats:

"Zero Trans Fat"-labeled packaged foods. The FDA guidelines only specify that there is less than ½ gram per serving.

Make sure that hydrogenated oils and partially hydrogenated oils are not in the ingredients.

Supermarket Pastries and Pre-Made Food. Donuts, bread items, corn dogs and many other unlabeled supermarket foods are in this category.

Restaurant food. Make sure you ask what restaurants are using for frying oil. Better yet, avoid fried foods when eating out.

Margarine and shortening. These have always been the worst offenders. Always check. Better yet...eat butter.

Snacks. Many crackers, cookies, and chips are still slipping in unhealthy amounts of trans-fats.

AVOID BAD FOODS

Take a quick look at your peanut butter, crackers, cookies and other favorites and make sure that there is none of the "bad" stuff. Remember, that labels may be misleading. Read the ingredients.

Know that donuts and other bakery items do contain trans fats. Gradually cut back on the amount of these items that you eat. Remember, if the fat doesn't get you, the sugar will. Most bakery breads still contain high fructose corn syrup.

BENEFITS:

- We are finally experiencing the freedom of knowing that the only truly "bad" fat is actually a "man-made" substance.

- Trans fats are slowly disappearing from our food chain. Avoid them and help make sure that they totally disappear.

- Eliminating trans fats is a major step in moving in the direction of healthy weight.

CHOOSE A HEALTHY BRAND PRODUCT AND KEEP USING IT

WEEK 7 - DAY 6

"I feed my body healthy fat to burn off stored fat."

HABIT 10: FUEL WITH LIPIDS FOR NORMAL BODY FUNCTIONS

Our goal today is to end our week of lipid lessons on a clear note. Our intention is to discuss fat burning (thermogenesis) and in doing so, it is always a temptation to talk about white fat and brown fat and adipose tissue and a whole bunch of other terms that may or may not have any real benefit at this point. So we'll attempt to resist that temptation and instead we'll focus our comments on ways that we can consume just the right amount of healthy fat each day so that our body will be turned on to burning the stored fat.

It goes pretty much like this. Those of us who carry extra fat, can literally turn that (brown) fat into an organ whose primary job is to waste excess calories obtained from food that is digested and assimilated, and already stored away as fat. Here are a few guidelines:

Carefully follow each of the suggestions from the previous lessons. **Never** again eat any "food-like" substances that contain trans fatty acids. Cut back on the amount of vegetable oils by reducing the amount of salad dressing and mayonnaise that you add to your meals.

Learn to find ways to supplement the amount of Omega-3 that you eat each day. In fact, consider adding one or two gel caps of a quality fish oil to your daily routine. One of our weight loss coaches insists that each of his clients consume at least 1000 mg of EPA and DHA in a fish oil capsule once a day. He is consistently one of our most successful coaches in terms of the satisfaction of the people that he is working with.

One of our best suggestions for weight loss is the Omega-3 fats found in flax. Look for cereals that contain flax seed or purchase a good quality flaxseed oil. If that does not sound good to you, try supplementing with capsules. One tablespoon of flaxseed oil equals about 12 capsules.

How did we do? Is this fat (lipid) stuff any more clear? As a team, we all agree that this can easily be the most confusing issue of this entire healthy weight discussion. We suggest that we all keep learning, that we all strive to keep an open mind, and that we continue to discuss this topic and learn together. Let's wrap up this week with a reminder of the good news.

There are only three food types. Just remember to enjoy lean, clean protein throughout the day, choose the colorful carbs, and enjoy the healthy forms of lipids in moderation. Here's a helpful tip borrowed from one of next week's lessons.....When you go to the store, avoid the stuff in boxes. Buy the real food around the outer edge of the store.

EAT HEALTHY FATS

Be creative. Start with olives or avocado. Find some fun ways to eat tasty mixed nuts and seeds. Learn about flax seed and chia seed. Remember that eggs are an excellent source of healthy fat.

Buy real, not processed and pasteurized, tasty cheese. Have some string cheese or some cubed cheese as a snack. Try a combination of cheddar cheese, almonds, and apple slices for a mini-meal.

BENEFITS

- Real whole food is the best source of healthy fats. The incredible, edible egg is a good example.

- It is not important to understand **how** this fat burning works. It is important to discover **that** it works.

THERE IS "FAT-BURNING" VALUE

IN EATING THE HEALTHY FATS

WEEK 7 - DAY 7

"Today is a break day."

HABIT 7: REFRESH TO STRENGTHEN YOUR COMMITMENT

We've saved some of the fun stuff for Week 8. You know, things like reading nutrition labels (and making sense out of all those numbers) and eating while you're "on the run".

Take a day off. In fact, take several days off. If you care to, look at the very back of the book. We have some interesting ideas on how you can stay "fresh", beat the stress, and find ways to continually renew your spirit and your energy.

REMEMBER...DON'T SWEAT THE SMALL STUFF

WEEK 8 - DAY 1

"I will form good habits and they will serve me."

HABIT 4: PLAN TO SUCCEED

It is time now to pause and to reassess where you are on your healthy eating pilgrimage. Each day you have been asked to "try on" a new healthy eating habit. Like "trying on" a new piece of clothing, you have been asked to get a feel for the new healthy eating habit; to figure out what it's like to do it throughout the day.

At this point, you have "tried on" ten new healthy eating habits including all of the food instructions we have just learned. Rather than focusing on the specifics, we want to start this preliminary evaluation by taking a look at the big picture. Let's start by asking ourselves a few key questions:

What have I learned about myself so far as it relates to healthy eating?

Has anything surprised me at this point, about myself as it relates to the habits?

"It has been harder than what I thought it would be to:

"It has been easier than what I thought it would be to:

The main new Healthy Eating concept or fact that I have learned is:

I'm still not sold on some things taught in this program. They include:

My motivation now as compared to when I started is: higher/lower.

My support system compared to when I started is: stronger/weaker?

The best thing I have going for me right now that will contribute to my success in eating more healthy is:

My biggest obstacle I face right now in eating more healthy is:

The one thing I've learned that will make the biggest difference in my life is:

REINFORCE THE TEN HABITS

Any behavior, practiced on a daily basis, becomes a habit. Are you learning to strengthen the Ten Habits in these vital areas to attain and maintain the level of health that you desire? It begins with your Why. Take at least five minutes today to explain what you are learning in these lessons to another person. Tell them your version of the benefits of maximum health.

Summarize each habit in a file or on a file card. Commit to reviewing the habits on a regular basis. Maybe tape a habit to the mirror you use in the morning to review it.

BENEFITS

- Healthy habits put into action lead to a desired state known as "Positive Addiction".

- Improvement in physical health quickly leads to a corresponding increase in mental health and well-being.

WE HAVE NOW SHARED THE 10 HABITS TO HEALTH

WEEK 8 - DAY 2

"I am learning to choose real foods over Franken-foods."

HABIT 5: NOURISH WITH REAL FOOD

A Franken-food is a popular term for a man-made or processed food-like substance. You know, like Frankenstein. We'll give a great list of real foods with which to begin. Here are 25 of the top foods that should always be on your list. We've even put them in alphabetical order.

1. Avocado
2. Barley
3. Beans
4. Beef (grass-fed)
5. Blueberries
6. Brown Rice
7. Chicken
8. Cinnamon
9. Citrus fruit
10. Dark chocolate
11. Eggs
12. Fish
13. Flax
14. Garlic
15. Green tea
16. Nuts and seeds
17. Oats
18. Olive Oil

19. Onion	23. Tomatoes
20. Quinoa	24. Wild Rice
21. Raspberries	25. Yogurt
22. Sprouts	26. *Still Learning*

Be sure to add your favorites as long as they are real foods. Where you find that you don't exactly agree, with what's on our list, keep an open mind and continue to learn. Remember that if the food has a long list of ingredients, you can probably live without it. As our friend, Michael Pollan, would say... "Don't eat anything that your great grandmother would not recognize as food."

REAL FOOD

Make a shopping list to plan for one shopping trip to the supermarket to buy only real food. Tomorrow we'll tell you more about how to do that.

Pick one category from this list above such as Beans. Make a commitment to learn more about how ways to prepare and enjoy that real food.

BENEFITS

- The powerful nutrients in these incredible whole foods were meant to be eaten just as they were grown, not as some scientist put them together in a laboratory.

- Eating foods as close to live as possible brings out the full amount of the flavor and the richness.

AS YOU CAN SEE ... IT'S ALL ABOUT FOOD

WEEK 8 - DAY 3

"I shop for real food around the periphery of the store."

HABIT 5: NOURISH WITH REAL FOOD

We once wrote a 16-page booklet on this subject. Even though our readers agreed that it was all important stuff, they said it was way too much information. Today we'll cover 5 main topics with several important ideas in each category.

- Do some planning. Make a list. Stick to it while at the store. Have a budget. Stock up when you find non-perishable items on sale. You've heard all of these before. Right? Do you practice what you know?

- Spend most of your time shopping around the outer edge (perimeter) of the store. Get to know the produce section...find out which day the fresh fruits and veggies arrive. Order fresh, thinly-sliced lean meats and cheeses at the "deli" section.

- Visit the "aisles" once a month (at most) for condiments, canned meats, some healthy cereals and crackers, spices, nuts, beans....you get the picture. Most of the stuff in the aisles is not real food...it is packaged and processed.

- The exception is the frozen section. Always have a good stock of your favorite vegetables and fruits in your freezer. Stay away from the packaged meals and the prepared food items. Most have too much added sugar and salt. Look for small, tasty ice cream treats. There are some with only about 100 calories for an evening snack.

- Slowly learn to make better choices. Later this week we'll talk about reading labels and knowing better what you are looking at. Here's our favorite tip in the cereal aisle.....The only cereal that is worth eating is on the top shelf. We promise.

SMART SHOPPING

Great eating begins with smart shopping. Spend an extra hour this week in shopping at the store using the concepts in this lesson, especially the tips in the first list above.

We saved this one for last. We know that you've heard this one. **Never** go grocery shopping when you are hungry.

BENEFITS

- When grocery shopping is a positive experience, rather than a "chore", you will find that you will take your time and often make better choices.

- There are dozens of ways to save money at the grocery store. Pick a favorite store and learn their practices about mark-downs and other types of savings.

WE EAT FOODS – WE DON'T EAT NUTRIENTS

WEEK 8 - DAY 4

"I choose healthy foods from any restaurant menu."

HABIT 5: NOURISH WITH REAL FOOD

If you are going to eat out, think about what you are eating the rest of the day so you can plan well and not get off your eating plan. For instance, think about the 3-hour guideline.

Always remember that restaurants are in the business of serving customers. Don't be afraid to ask for items specially prepared the way you want them. Begin with these practical suggestions:

- Don't tempt yourself. Remove the chips, peanuts, or bread after you've had a small amount, or you may even choose to leave them off the table altogether. Avoid mindless nibbling.

- Get exactly what you want by ordering each item separately (a la carte). For example, one chicken enchilada easy-on-the-sauce, side salad, and fruit desert instead of the #8 enchilada plate with rice, beans, sour cream, guacamole, etc.

- Order regular portion sizes instead of the jumbo sizes now common. Try an appetizer, half an entrée, or share a meal with a friend and order an extra side salad. Ask for half the entrée to be wrapped up to go, even before the food is brought to the table.

- Ask how dishes are prepared and the have them do it your way do it your way: grill the chicken, steam the vegetables, bring sauces and salad dressings on the side, put just a dollop of cream sauce on the pasta primavera and extra grilled vegetables.

- Go easy on or preferably even eliminate the alcohol. It's high calorie, has few nutrients, and certainly can weaken your will power.

EAT OUT BUT EAT HEALTHY

Do an internet search and look for restaurants in your area that serve healthy food. Try a new place this week.

When your lunch sandwich is more than you can eat, take ½ back to the office. It makes a great mid-afternoon snack.

BENEFITS

- You can still enjoy your favorite eating places and many of your favorite foods. Learn to make healthy choices.

- You'll enjoy your meal more by remembering two of our previous habits. Don't wash down your food with beverages and remember to chew your food thoroughly.

USE THE MENU AS A REFERENCE - ORDER FOOD TO YOUR LIKING

WEEK 8 - DAY 5

"I am learning to choose fast food that is really good food."

HABIT 5: NOURISH WITH REAL FOOD

First, it can be done. Not all fast food meals are necessarily unhealthy.

Sandwich choices

- Order the smallest burger available, and ask for extra lettuce, tomato and onion. Remember that cheese adds an extra 100 calories and 8 to 10 grams of fat.

- Go light on the extras. Mayo, sautéed mushrooms and bacon all add an average of 90 calories and 8 grams of fat. Use mustard, which has zero fat, instead of mayo with 100 calories per tablespoon.

- A fried chicken or fish sandwich has as much fat and calories as an extra-large burger. Instead, go for the grilled, un-breaded option.

- Use special sauces or tartar sauce sparingly. Having them served on the side will help you consume smaller quantities.

Salad suggestions

- Order a salad with grilled chicken (no breading). Use low-calorie or nonfat dressing. Regular dressing will add over 200 calories and 15 grams of fat. Avoid Chinese noodles, croutons, bacon and tortilla chips.

Be careful with the beverage

- One large 32-ounce soda has as much as 425 calories and 26 teaspoons of sugar (high fructose corn syrup). Order water, unsweetened iced tea or low fat milk instead.

- A small shake can have as much as 360 calories and 10 grams of fat. This is not a good choice.

Fries and onion rings

- A small order of fries or onion rings can have as much as 200 calories or more and over 10 grams of fat. If you really want a taste, consider sharing with someone. Otherwise, substitute a side salad with low-cal dressing.

Other healthy options

- Chili, with or without onions and a small amount of shredded cheese.

- Fruit cups or a yogurt parfait.

- Wraps or pitas with turkey, roast beef or ham. Add extra lettuce, tomatoes or other veggies, and go easy on the dressings, mayo and sauces.

MORE ABOUT EATING OUT

Notice that we do not talk about the deli sandwich places as fast food. With all of the fresh vegetable and bread choices, the sub places are almost always a better choice.

Avoid the typical fast food place when you are extremely hungry. Grab a full serving of water and do your best to find an alternative place to have your meal.

BENEFITS

- Choosing the "fast food" place for a quick snack instead of a meal, allows you the time to find a more nutritious place to eat.

- Most of the items on a fast food menu are good examples of "what not to eat".

DO NOT EAT FOOD WHILE IN THE CAR.

AVOID FOOD THAT HAS BEEN SERVED THROUGH A WINDOW

- MICHAEL POLLAN

Week 8 - Day 6

"I learn what I can about packaged foods by reading the labels."

HABIT 5: NOURISH WITH REAL FOOD

There are a couple of very important pieces of information on the nutrition labels of packaged foods. If you are interested in learning as much as you can about this topic, we have added a link at the end of this message for you to get a complete description. Here's a quick focus on the most useful facts:

Serving size and number of servings: Remember our previous example of the bottle of iced tea. It contained 2 and ½ servings. A bag of trail mix may list 135 calories, but the bag contains 6 servings (810 calories). A can of soup may show 735 grams of sodium but contains 3 servings (a full daily allowance of salt). It is just as important to know the number of servings in the container as the serving size.

Calories and calories from fat: The real key here is to remember that the **number of calories is listed as calories per serving.** Remember that bottle of tea was only about 120 calories per serving but each bottle was two and one-half servings per bottle... Remember that the whole bottle was equivalent to 16 teaspoons of sugar and nearly 300 calories. The same is true for the listings about the different forms of fat. This is where the fat in salad dressings can get us into trouble if we consume more than a serving.

Listing for each key nutrient: You'll notice that each of the three food types is listed in some detail, and the label also contains information about cholesterol and sodium. Again, if you are watching either or both of these nutrients, remember what is listed is per serving. The two biggest challenges with packaged and processed food is added salt and sugar. See why we love live foods?

Every current food label breaks down the amount of fat, carbohydrates (listings for sugar and fiber), and protein per serving. While we have never emphasized calorie counting, healthy eating requires that you continue to watch the balance of your foods and know what each nutrient provides. Check our website for a link to the FDA information on food labels.

READ TO BE WISE

Pick a couple of cans or boxes of food that you buy most often. What is the serving size? Is that about the amount that you usually eat? Look especially for information that you may not have known.

The next time you are at the supermarket, spend some time looking at bread information. Notice especially the ingredients listed first (the flour). Is it whole grain? Do you see words like enriched or fortified? Is there any high fructose corn syrup? For many of us, bread and other bakery items provide a good place for us to start learning a lot more about our food.

BENEFITS

- A recent study showed that most of us know a lot more about the software that we load on our computers than we do about what is in the food that we eat. You can do better than that. Begin with this simple course and continue to increase your knowledge of food.

- Your body will love you for it. The benefits are many and they are life-long. Remember your Why.

IN TIME ALL FOOD LABELS WILL BECOME MORE ACCURATE
AND MORE USEFUL
LET'S WORK TOGETHER TO MAKE SURE

WEEK 8 - DAY 7

CELEBRATE!

HABIT 7: REFRESH TO STRENGTHEN YOUR COMMITMENT

Can you believe it? A lifetime of healthy eating awaits as you now continue to form and apply these habits. We're so excited that you've stuck with the program and made it all the way to this point. We're going to suggest a few days off and then a quick review. For those who are really serious about this health stuff, we will follow this week with a popular module included in every course that we have offered. You know, the activity that carries the deep philosophical title **WHAT NOW?**

Come back in a day or two and complete the final exercise. We've also added a special bonus at the end of the book to help you keep fresh and beat the stress in your life.

"CELEBRATE WHAT YOU WANT TO SEE MORE OF."

THOMAS PETERS

WHAT NOW?

THINGS TO KNOW ABOUT CHANGING HABITS

Your whole system is going through change - When changing habits as we've been working at, it's sometimes hard to see things clearly. Realize that you have been putting your entire emotional and physical system through change. It often distorts the way we feel and the way we think. Try to SEE what you are doing RIGHT. We often times don't give ourselves credit for what we are doing right/accomplishing and we often deny admitting some of our obstacles.

- **The key to lifestyle change is to build success upon success** and to realistically adapt the new behavior into your lifestyle. Don't set yourself up to fail by taking on too big of a chunk. We don't want you to be on the "yo-yo" nutrition program, on it one month, off it the next. That is not a healthy way to live.

- **Look realistically at yourself and your life** - We want to encourage you to see things/yourself as they really are…many programs just try to get you to "talk yourself into" thinking that you can do it; using shear willpower; changing your "self-talk" and reciting affirmations to motivate yourself to do what you have a hard time doing. We don't think these strategies have lasting effect. We have confidence that the best way to help you succeed is to see yourself clearly and accurately as it relates to changing these lifestyle behaviors.

- **Consider your belief system** - The best way to change any habit is not through gimmicks, but rather by adopting a new belief system.

- **Ask yourself:** which method has the best chance of working over the long haul:

- **Continuously telling** yourself that you can do it, using shear will power, or

- **Really believing** it is the right thing for you to do?

DEVELOPING SUCCESSFUL BELIEF SYSTEMS

Hopefully, you choose the second answer to the previous question. Adopting a belief about something, learning to value a healthy habit, is the best way for lasting change. Let's talk about how you learn to value your health in such a way that it will lead to permanent positive healthy lifestyle change. Learning to value anything (developing a belief system) and particularly your health typically goes through a process as described below:

1. A spark is lit – This can come about for various reasons, perhaps a comment was made to you about the way you look,

your doctor scared you, you read something, you saw a friend succeed, etc.

2. Experimentation with the change – Once the spark is lit, most people start to dabble in the new healthy behavior. They "try it on", see what it feels like to do it and see what effect it has on their lives.

3. Finding success – usually through trial and error, if the person comes upon success, the belief system starts to take hold. They are starting to determine that the healthy behavior may work for them, that they can do it. This is why it is important to set yourself up for success by making your goals achievable.

4. Motivation increases – Not only does the belief start to take hold, but motivation increases. Remember, success breeds success. Set yourself up for success.

5. Belief grows – belief and motivation go hand in hand. As you have more success, motivation increases and belief follows.

6. More success follows – Once motivation increases, more success follows. The person may find themselves adding new healthy behaviors. It starts to become a lifestyle

7. Validation and integration of Belief – Once success takes hold, the person starts to validate their belief. They look for ways to confirm that what they are doing is good and right for them. It starts to take hold in their heart and becomes a part of them. The belief become integrated into "who they are". They identify with the behavior as part of them; "I'm a healthy person."

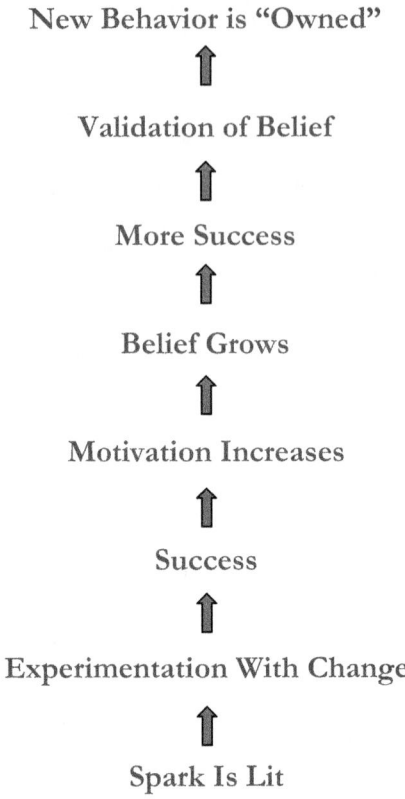

New Behavior is "Owned"

⇑

Validation of Belief

⇑

More Success

⇑

Belief Grows

⇑

Motivation Increases

⇑

Success

⇑

Experimentation With Change

⇑

Spark Is Lit

True, permanent change only happens when a belief system has been adopted. As it relates to healthy eating, we need to ask ourselves:

What do I really believe when it comes to the importance of healthy eating in my life and my family's life"?

Why am I doing this?

Do I really "buy-into" the idea that healthy eating will make much of a difference in my life?

Do I really care about my health and vitality at this point in my life?

We are asking you to go through an honest, thoughtful appraisal of where you are related to these questions. The reason most people go on "yo-yo" diets is because they never get to the point of **believing** in the healthy lifestyle change. We want to help you get this issue out into the open so that you are not a casualty to the "yo-yo" lifestyle. Instead, we want you to form the habits of healthy eating and a healthy lifestyle.

AND SO, WE'D LIKE TO SAY GOOD NIGHT

We have made the commitment that our goal is to get healthy so we can lose some unwanted weight. We've been together for some time now, and we know that you've begun to experience some real success. When you are ready for a substantial "boost" in your program, we have a refreshing idea to share with you as a way of saying Thank You for spending this time with us: **Turn off the television or computer an hour earlier each evening and go to bed.**

The majority of us today are getting too little good, rejuvenating sleep. We've learned a lot about the habits related to healthy eating and drinking. It's clearer now that certain food and drinks are contributing to our health issues. Too much sitting instead of being active is also definitely a part of the reason why overweight is now common. But studies suggest that a lack of sleep may make weight loss and weight control more of a challenge than it needs to be by altering our metabolism, as well as "messing with" our eating and activity patterns.

Changes in hormone levels have been linked to sleep deprivation in several studies. One hormone, cortisol, regulates metabolism of sugar, protein, fat, minerals and water. Physical or emotional stress raises cortisol levels. Lack of sleep has also been shown to raise levels of his "fat-storage" hormone at certain times of the day.

Second, higher levels of insulin, a condition known as insulin resistance, have also been linked to a shortage of sleep in several recent studies. Excess cortisol could be the link here as well. Since insulin not only controls blood sugar, but also promotes fat storage, extra insulin makes weight loss more difficult.

Because increasing stress levels are impacting so many of us today, research is being conducted in order to validate the hormonal changes observed. But even without any hormonal impact, sleep deprivation can promote weight gain by affecting our behavior. Here's what we mean...When people low on sleep find their energy dropping throughout the day, many turn to food for a pickup. The short-term rise in blood sugar gives a more energetic feeling, but unfortunately, the extra calories are not needed by the body at that time and end up being stored as body fat.

Furthermore, the most appealing foods when we feel low on energy are often sweets or refined carbohydrates with low nutrient density. If sleep deprivation causes insulin resistance, over consuming these types of carbohydrates will be especially problematic.

There's even more distressing news about this lack of sleep stuff. Not only is it easy to take in excess calories when sleep deprived. For many people, calorie burning decreases when we are exhausted. If your extra waking hours are spent in sedentary activities at a desk or computer or in front of the TV, you're not burning many more calories than when asleep.

And when sleep deprived, people are often too tired to exercise. Or if they do manage to exercise, they work out less intensely than usual. For example, a rested person may walk two miles in a half-hour, while someone more fatigued may go much less. The tired person would burn fewer calories, despite walking just as long.

Sleep experts recommend as close a possible to eight hours of sleep each night for most adults. Yet the latest data from the National Sleep Foundation suggests that Americans average just under seven hours during the workweek. In fact, a third of adults reportedly sleep no more than six-and-a-half hours nightly.

Shutting off the TV and logging off the computer an hour earlier each evening means an hour less possible munching time. Turning in earlier could also shift your metabolism to make weight control easier. It will definitely leave you with more energy to exercise. So with that we say "Good night."

HABIT 7: REFRESH TO STRENGTHEN YOUR COMMITMENT

ABOUT THE AUTHORS

Ron and Julie Meiss are the managing directors of the Center for Nutritional Science (C4NS). Founded in 1996 as an independent, science-based advocate for better nutrition and maximum health, C4NS is dedicated to clearing the confusion and improving communication as it relates to individual health.

Ron is a retired business executive who left the corporate rat-race at age 50 in pursuit of the elusive answers to nutrition, weight-loss and improved health. Julie became a client of C4NS in January, 2010 as a participant in the DOCTOR'S PLAN for Healthy Eating. They were married in October, 2010 and reside in Phoenix, AZ.

The mission of the Center is to provide a safe pathway for persons who are seeking to achieve a healthy weight. The premise is to correct the thinking that a person needs to attempt to lose weight in the search for better health. 15 years and thousands of clients have clearly shown that the more logical approach is to "get healthy and (then) lose weight". Each of the learning systems provided by C4NS is guided by this sensible, science-based philosophy.

Ron holds Master's degrees in Counseling and in Human Relations from Webster University and is the author and publisher of more than 40 personal development systems. Julie earned her RN degree in 1974 and serves as the clinical director of the Boswell Eye Institute in Sun City, AZ. She is the creator and the director of the Partner division of The Center for Nutritional Science.

Ron & Julie Meiss